Nursing The Journey.

Written by Vivienne Graves, DNP, APRN, FNP-BC

Welcome to the wonderful world of nursing. The journey will only sometimes be smooth or pleasant, but it will be one of your most rewarding and fulfilling experiences.

**"Press forward. Do not stop or linger in your journey, but strive for the mark set before you."-
George Whitefield**.

My name is Vivienne Graves, and I have been in nursing for over 30 years. I have been an Advanced Practice Nurse for 25 years. The purpose of this Novice Nurse guide is to provide you with valuable tips and advice on how to start this journey and transition from a student novice to a nurse.

"Faith is taking the first step even when you don't see the whole staircase." -Martin Luther King Jr.

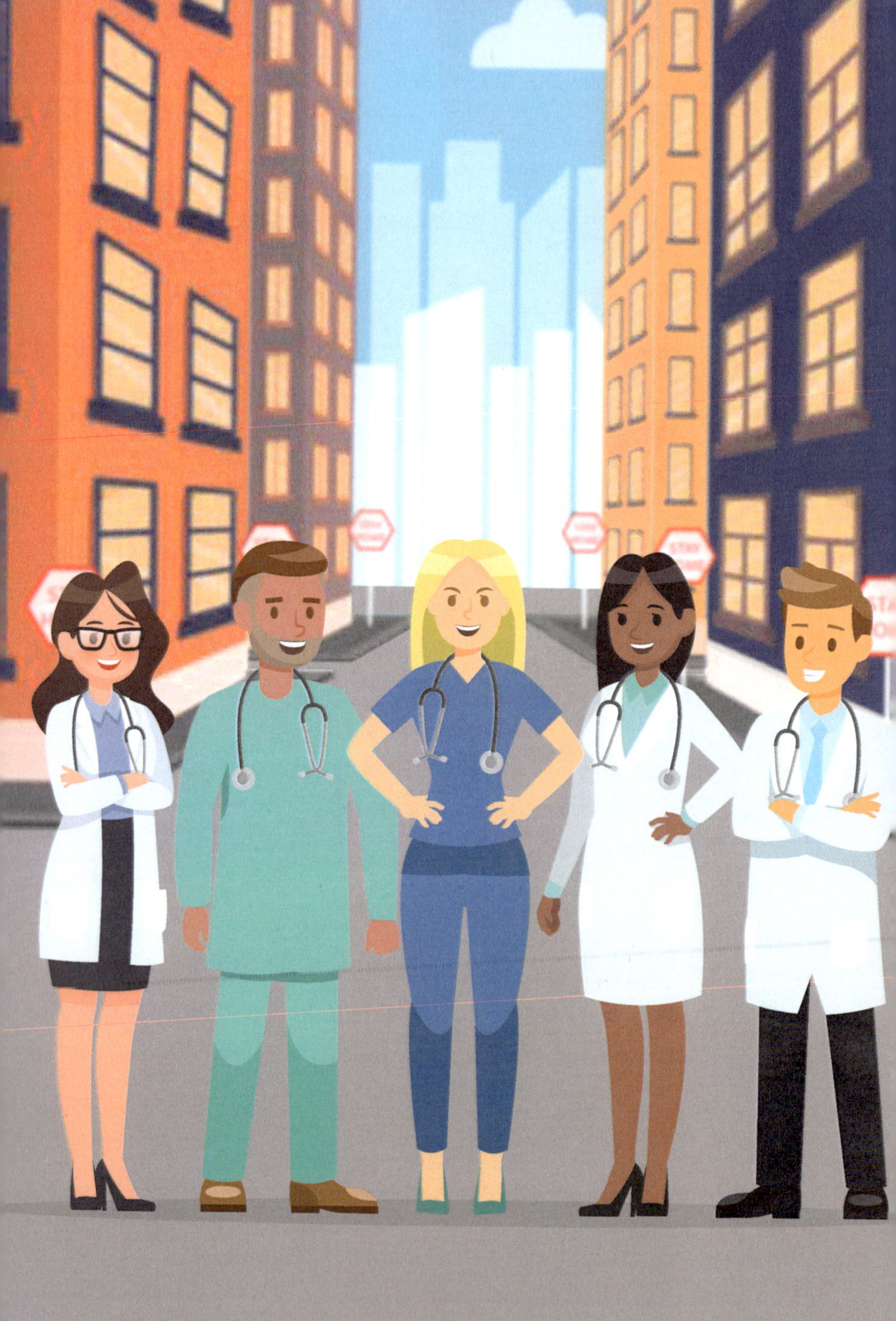

The first step can be scary and feel like an unknown territory, but you are ready; you have trained long and hard for this moment. Let us Begin!

1.   Community
Find or Establish a safe community of your peers. Seek out mentorship. Find a mentor Nurse you feel comfortable with.

2.   Communication
First and foremost, you must have good communication skills to communicate effectively with your patients, their family physicians' other nurses, and staff. Advance your communication skills by using self-help books and social media communications training. Use respectful language and always be socially aware and culturally sensitive.Ask questions; it is better to see clarification than make mistakes.

3.   Time Management
Organize your shifts, prioritize your tasks, and know what can wait versus what needs immediate attention. Learn how to triage and prioritize. Stay organized and have a system for your notes, task lists, and supplies. An organized nurse is the most efficient.

4.   Safety
Promote a safe environment where to practice. Prioritize safety by double-checking your physical assessment,medications, procedures, and fall risk. Always double-check medications. The safety of your patients is a top priority.

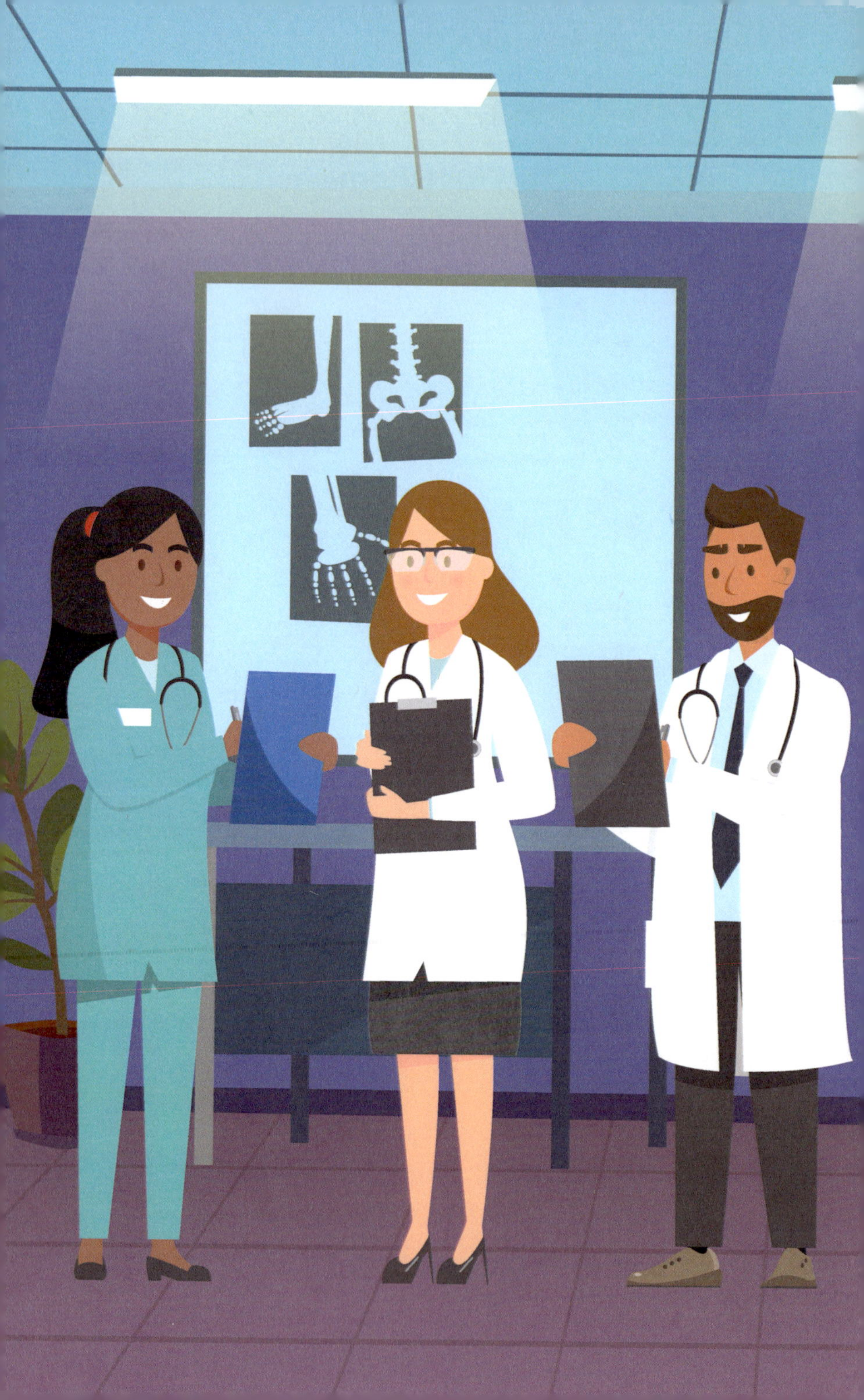

5. Sharpen your Basic Nursing Skills

Become an expert in proper hand hygiene, vital signs, recording vital signs, recording accurate intake and output, performing accurate physical assessments and medication administration, bed baths and hygiene, wound care and dressing, mobility, and positioning. Seek confirmation from your mentors when doing standard procedures like giving injections. Catheter insertion and care, nasogastric tube insertion and care, and tracheostomy care basics.

6. Work as a Team
Work as a team and encourage others to do so. Ask for help when needed. Be a supportive colleague and understand different roles in your working environment.

7. Continual Learning
Seek feedback, observe experienced nurses, and constantly research and read up on medical conditions and procedures. Complete your professional continuing education requirements on time. Advance your formal education, earn additional certifications, and learn new skills. Join professional organizations. Reflect on your practice regularly and evaluate your strengths and areas for improvement. With experience comes confidence. Believe in your ability to learn and care for patients.

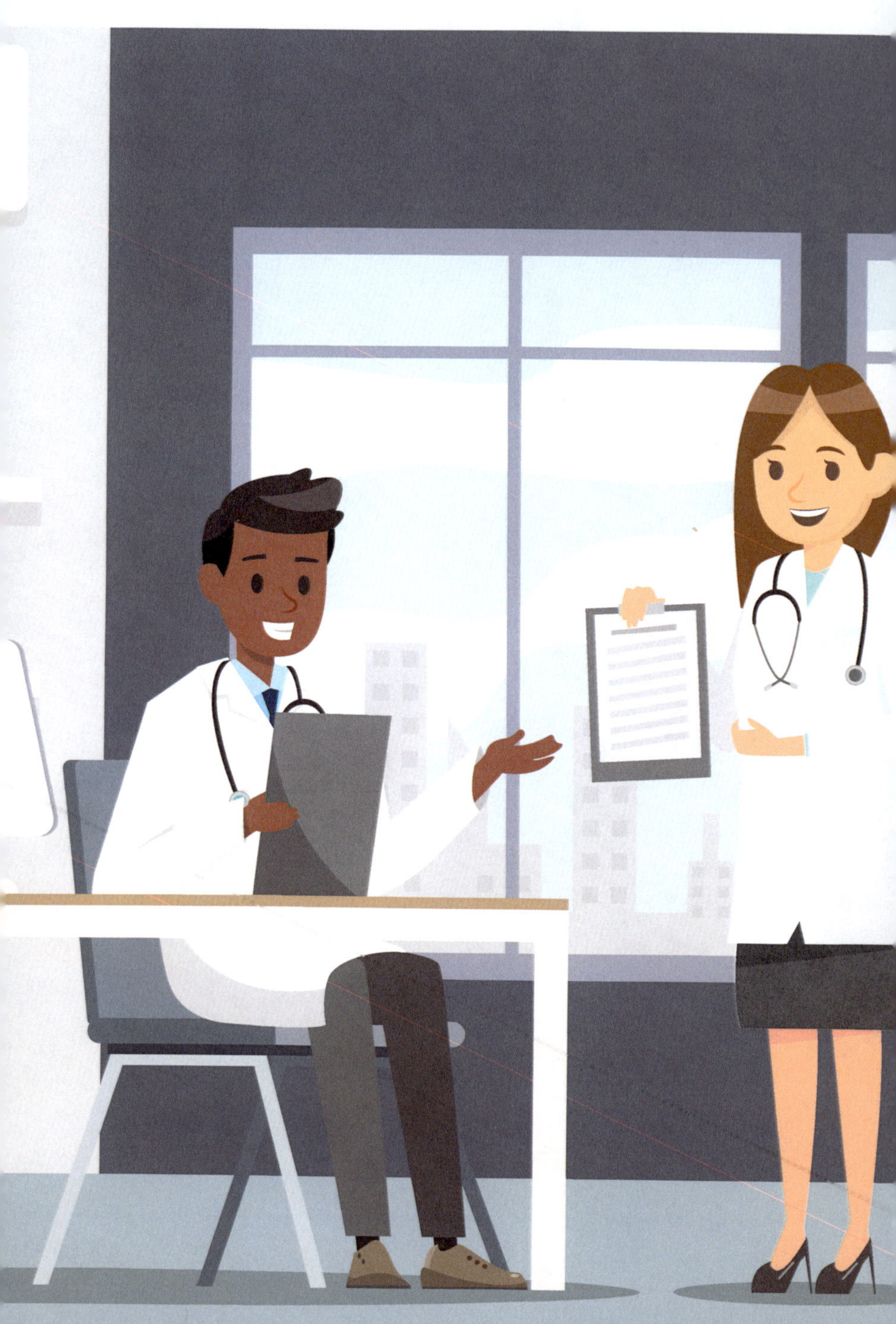

8. Self-care - Balance work and Personal lifePractice self-care to prevent burnout by eating healthy, exercising regularly, and getting adequate sleep. Be a supportive colleague and surround yourself with supportive peers and mentors. Learn techniques and methods of coping with complex patients and family situations. Take vacations and time off. Spend time caring for and being with family and friends.

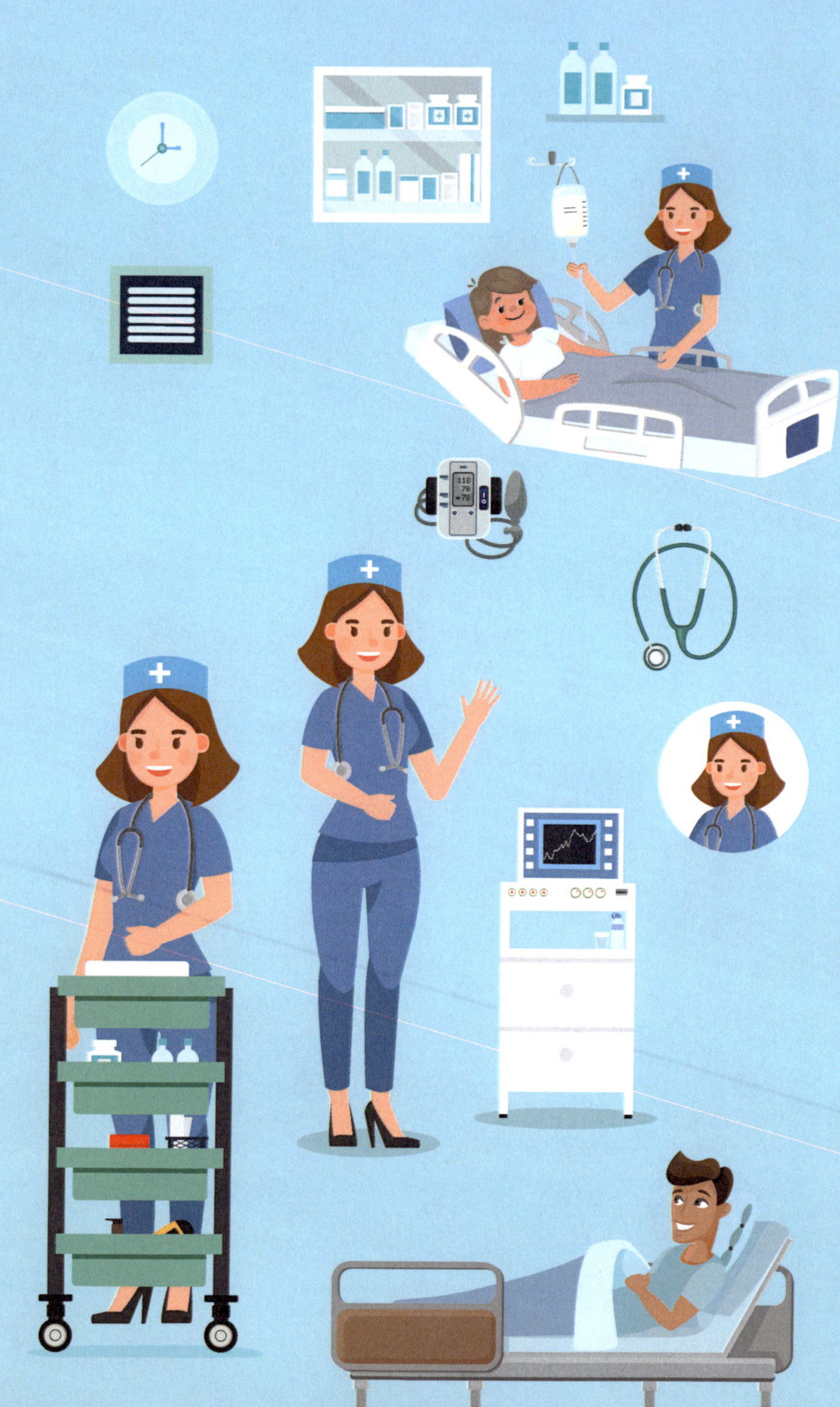

Tips on Time Management for Novice Nurses:

•Create a shift to-do list and prioritize tasks based on
 urgent patient needs. Cross items off as completed.
  Chunk similar tasks together
 [vital signs, assessment, medication] to work efficiently.

•Allow extra time for new/ complex procedures and
 patients until skills are mastered.

•Learn shortcuts like frequently accessed areas on
 charts or supply locations.

• Say no to unnecessary tasks outside your scope and
  stay on top of patients' responsibilities.

•Pace yourself, and don't hesitate to ask for help if you
 run behind. Communicate delays appropriately.

•Meal and break times are non-negotiable for
 recharging. Schedule ahead when possible.

•Come prepared with the necessary supplies and
 documents ready for each shift.

•Streamline documentation by entering as you go
 when able instead of batching at the end of the shift.

•Learn from experienced nurses what can be safely
 delegated in a pinch.

•Be punctual arriving and leaving shifts and meetings to
 respect others' time.

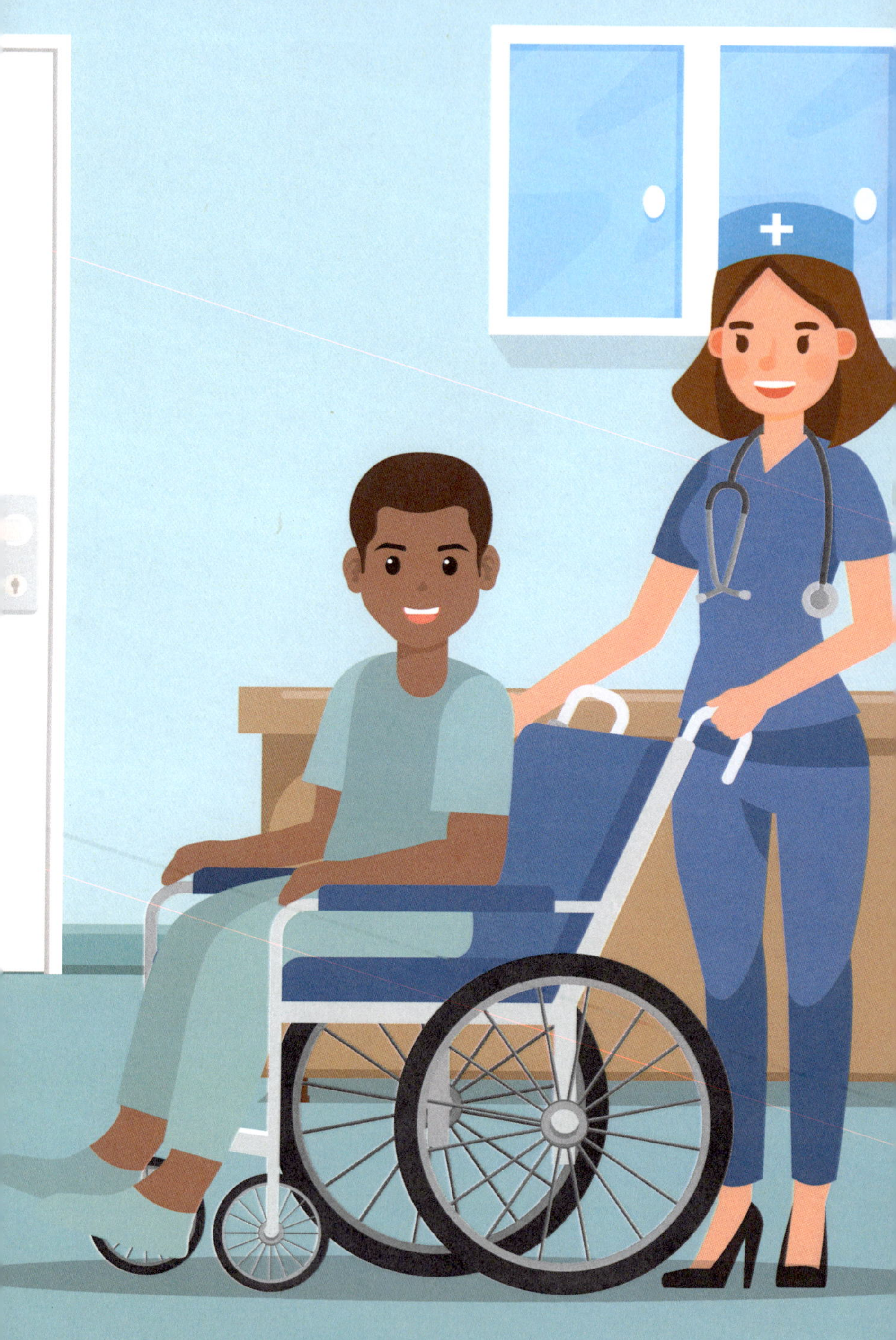

- Realistic scheduling allows time for unforeseen issues like emergencies or procedure delays.

- With practice and repetition, time management skills will improve. Don't be too hard on yourself as a new nurse.

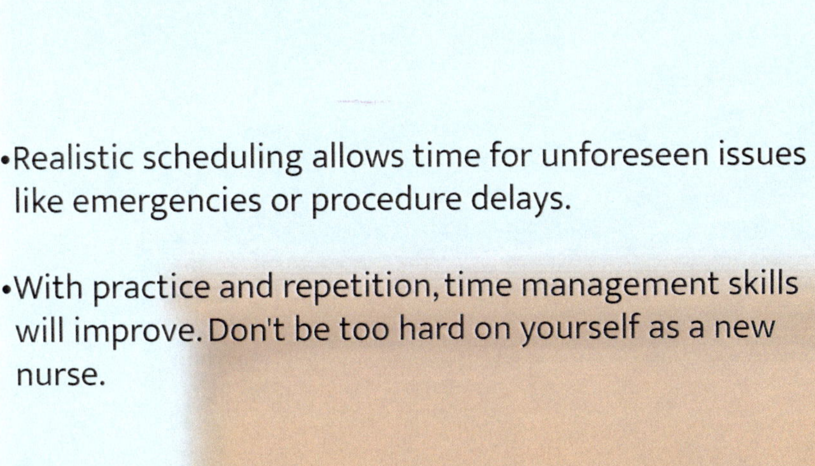

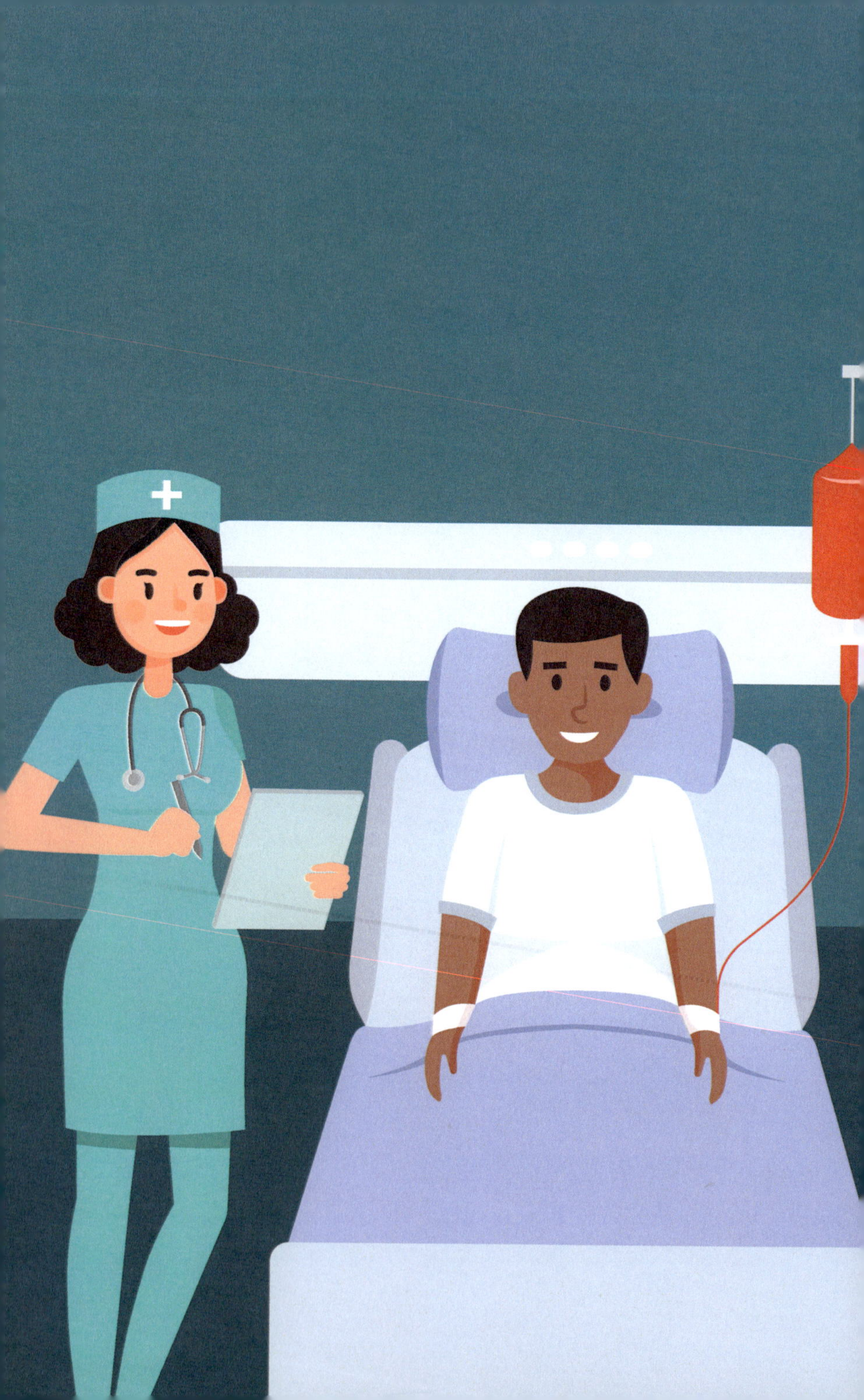

The difference between ordinary and extraordinary is that little extra" -Jimmy Johnson.

Whispers of Wellness: A Symphony in Nursing Exploration

Patient Advocacy & Empathy

Patient advocacy and empathy form the heart of nursing practice, embodying the compassionate essence of healthcare. As a nurse, your role extends beyond the clinical to champion the rights and needs of your patients, ensuring their well-being and fostering a trusting relationship.

Advocating for Patients' Needs & Rights

Advocacy involves being a vocal supporter for your patients, standing as a stalwart defender of their rights and ensuring they receive the highest standard of care. This extends to communicating with interdisciplinary teams, ensuring patients' voices are heard, and navigating bureaucratic processes on their behalf.

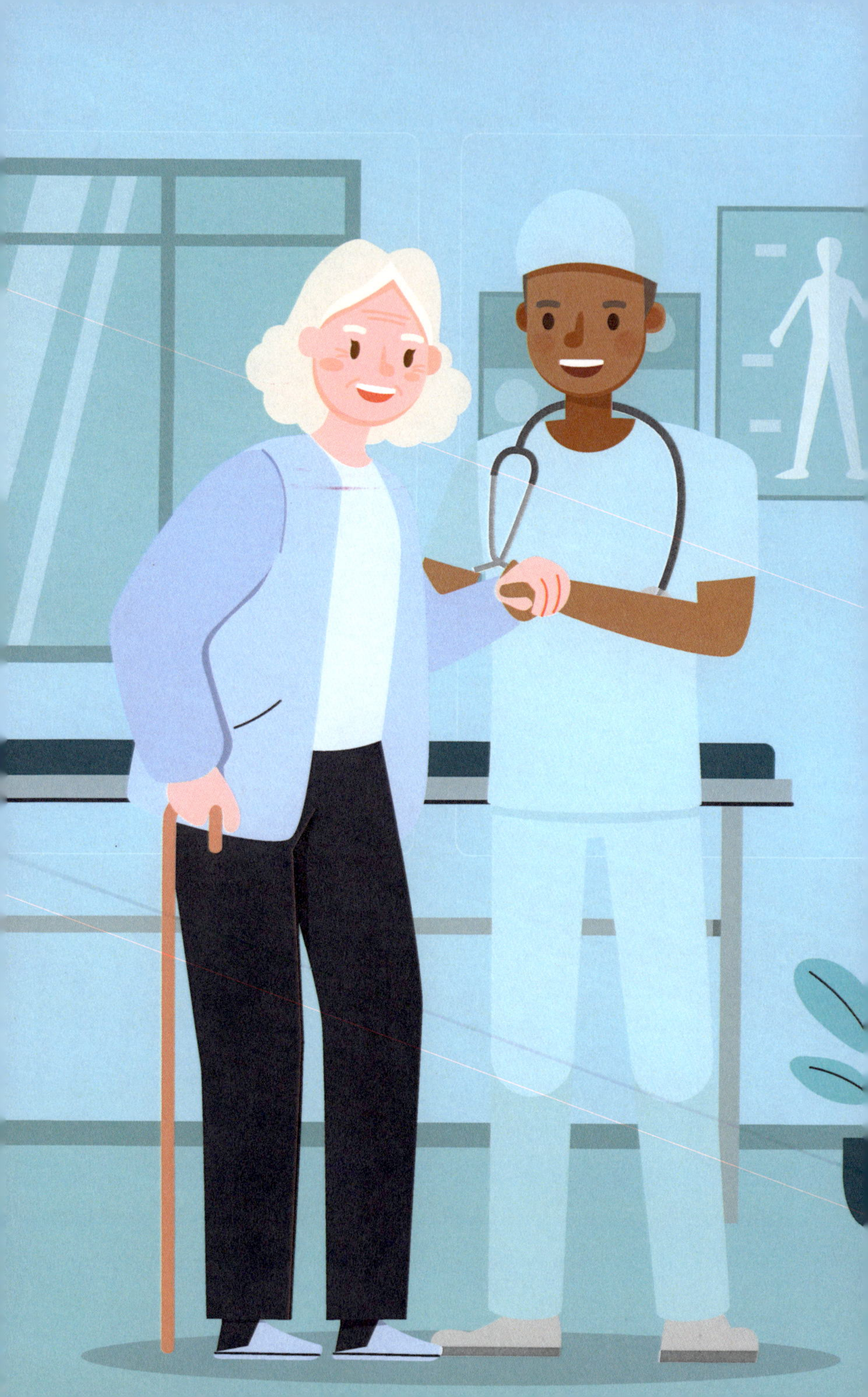

Constant attention by a good nurse may be just as important as a major operation by a surgeon.
" —Dag Hammarskjöld, Swedish economist and diplomat.

The Impact of Empathy on Patient Care

Empathy is the cornerstone of effective healthcare. By understanding and sharing patients' emotions, you can forge connections that transcend the purely clinical. Genuine empathy has the power to produce a profound impact. It humanizes the nursing experience and illustrates empathy's effectiveness on patients and caregivers.

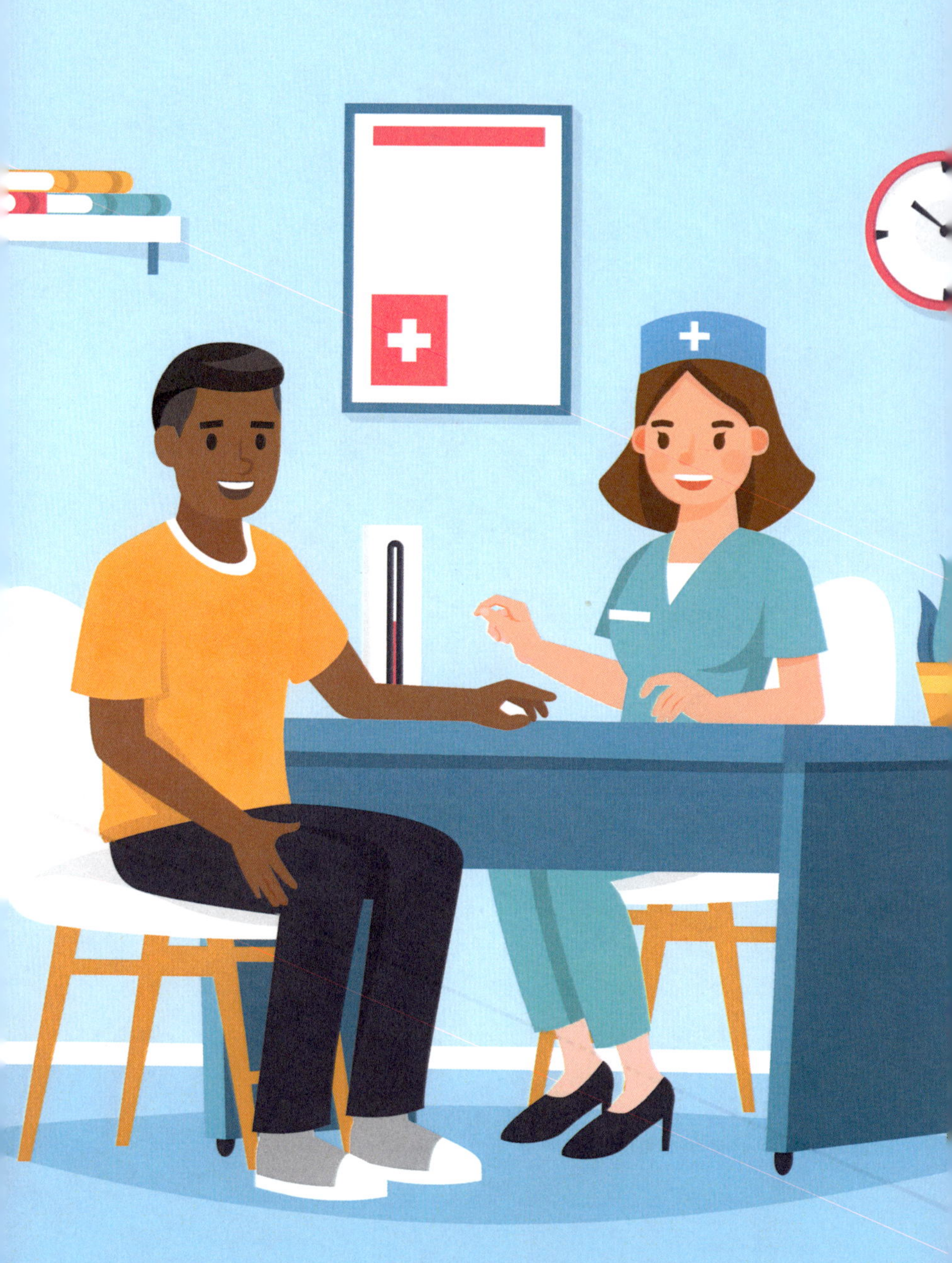

Effective Communication in Challenging Times

Communication during difficult moments is an art that nurses must master. Here are some practical tips to help you master this art:

Establish a Comfortable Environment:
- Ensure privacy and create a quiet, comfortable space for the conversation.
- Minimize interruptions to foster an environment conducive to open communication.

Active Listening:
- Demonstrate active listening by giving your full attention to the patient.
- Make appropriate verbal and non-verbal cues, such as nodding or occasional affirmations, to convey your engagement.

Maintain Eye Contact:
- Eye contact is a powerful non-verbal cue that conveys empathy and attentiveness.
- Strike a balance by maintaining eye contact without making the patient uncomfortable.

Employ Open-Ended Questions:
- Encourage patients to express their thoughts and concerns by asking open-ended questions.
- Instead of yes or no answers, these questions invite patients to share more about their feelings and experiences.

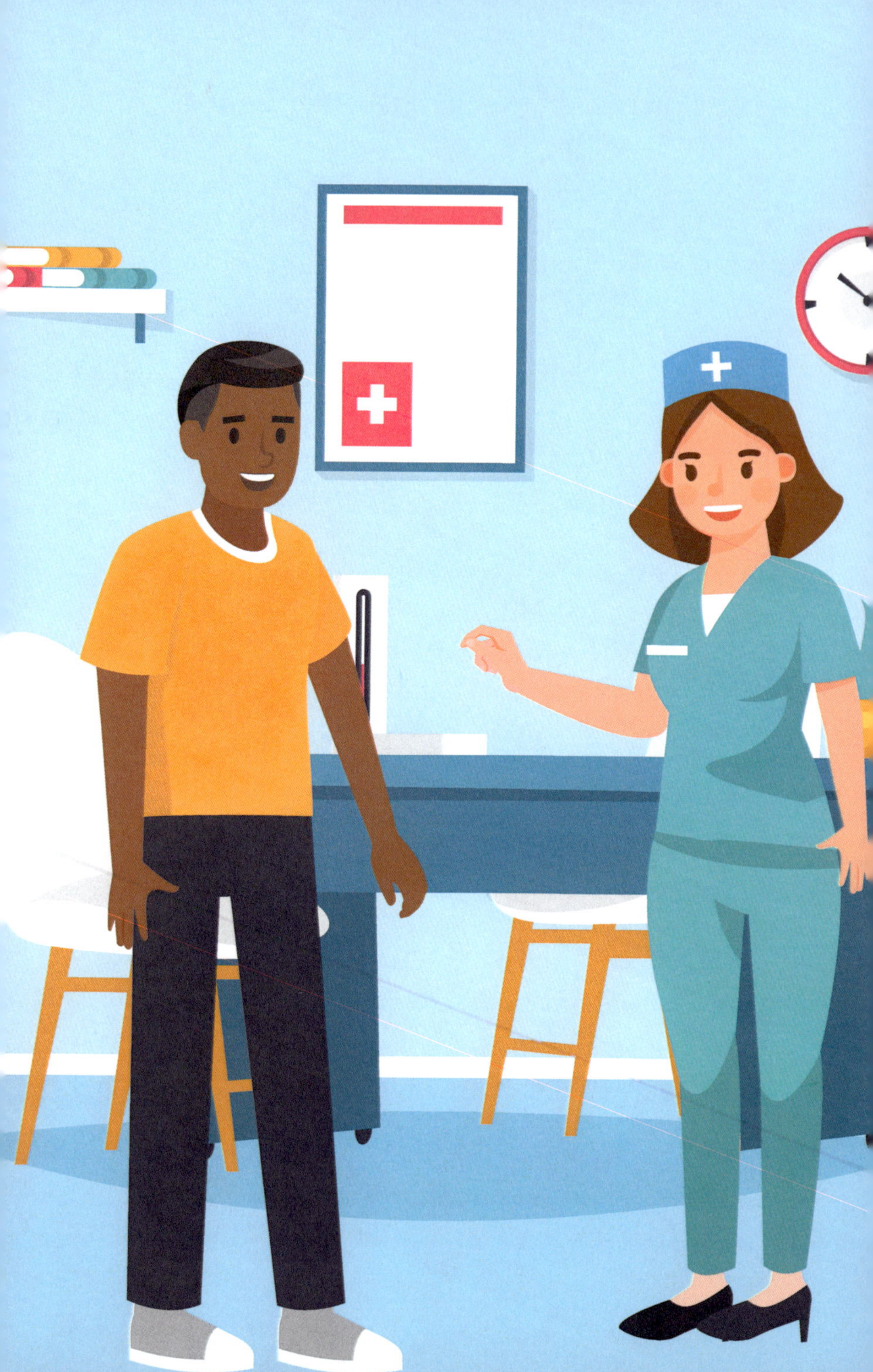

Use Empathetic Language:
- Choose words carefully to convey empathy and understanding.
- Acknowledge the patient's emotions and validate their feelings to create a supportive atmosphere.

Be Mindful of Non-Verbal Cues:
- Pay attention to your own non-verbal cues to ensure they align with your verbal communication.
- A compassionate facial expression and open body language contribute to a comforting atmosphere.

Avoid Interrupting:
- Allow the patient to express themselves fully without interruption.
- Once they have shared their thoughts, respond thoughtfully and considerately.

Summarize and Clarify:
- Periodically summarize what the patient has shared to demonstrate understanding.
- Seek clarification if needed to ensure an accurate interpretation of their concerns.

Express Empathy and Understanding:
- Verbally express empathy by acknowledging the challenges the patient is facing.
- Use phrases like "I understand" or "I can see this is difficult for you."

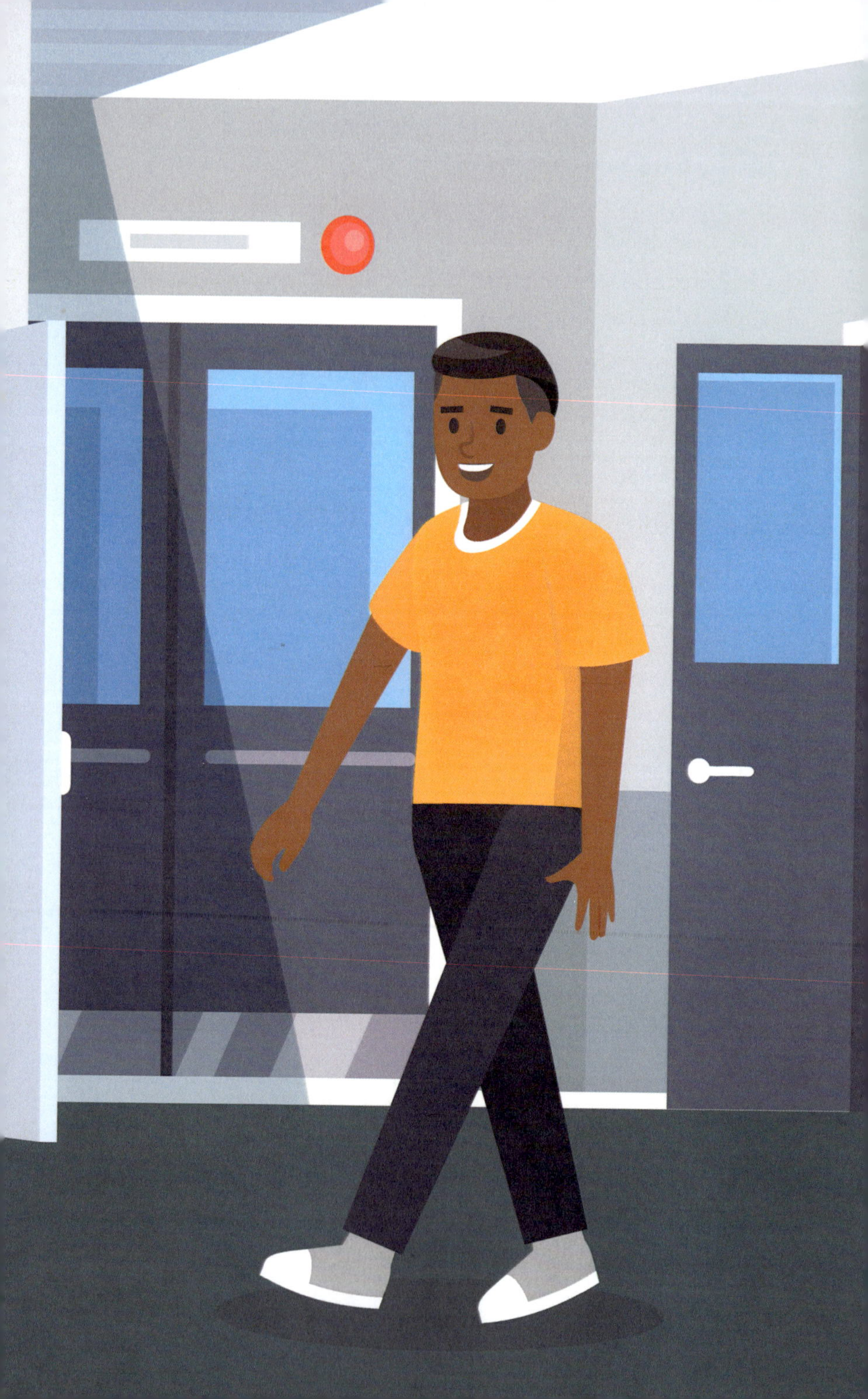

Offer Support and Solutions:
- Collaboratively explore potential solutions or support systems.
- Communicate the next steps or actions, ensuring patients feel informed and involved in their care.

Ever heard of shared decision-making? It's like teaming up with patients to create care plans that feel just right. Respecting their choices, keeping them in the loop, and making sure they feel like the heroes of their healthcare journey—it's all part of the friendly game plan. It's not just about improving the quality of care; it's about making the healthcare system feel like a friendly chat with an old pal.

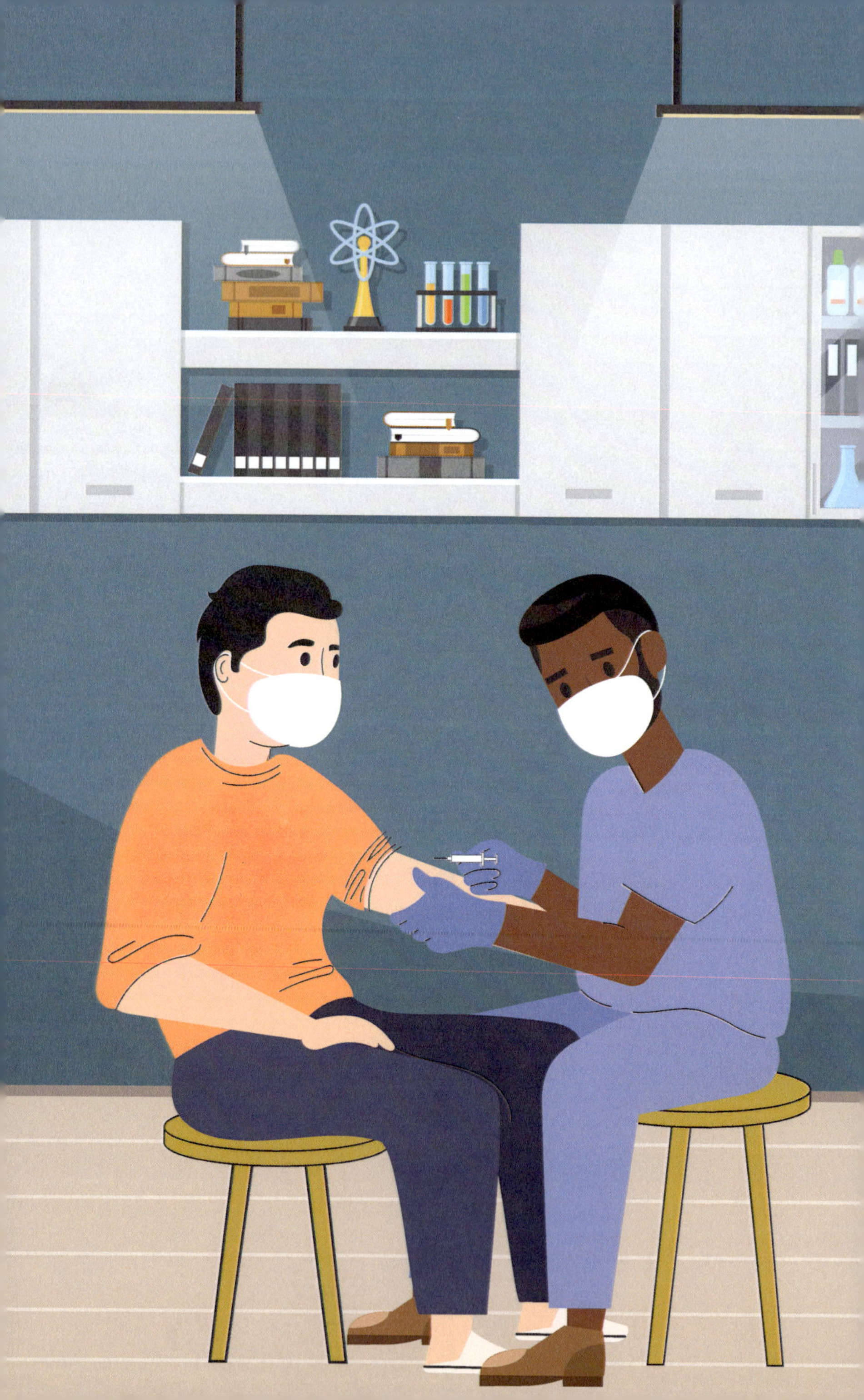

Tips on how to Develop Critical Nursing Skills:

- Ask questions to understand the root cause/ pathology behind the patient's condition or issues.

- Look up diseases/ procedures you're unfamiliar with to learn signs/ symptoms and standard treatment plans. Compare a patient's presentation to what is expected based on their diagnosis or lab results. Consider alternative possibilities.

- Observe experienced nurses closely. Watch how they assess patients, communicate with physicians and other staff, handle emergencies, and more.

- Develop both your technical skills and soft skills. Ask questions, period. Be bold and ask nurses, physicians, and other care team members questions about what you observe and how to handle different situations. This shows initiative.

- Volunteer for additional training opportunities. Look for classes, simulations, and programs that allow you to practice skills in a low-pressure environment.

- Practice skills regularly. Continually refine skills like physical assessment, medication administration, and wound care. Even during downtime at work period, repetition is essential.

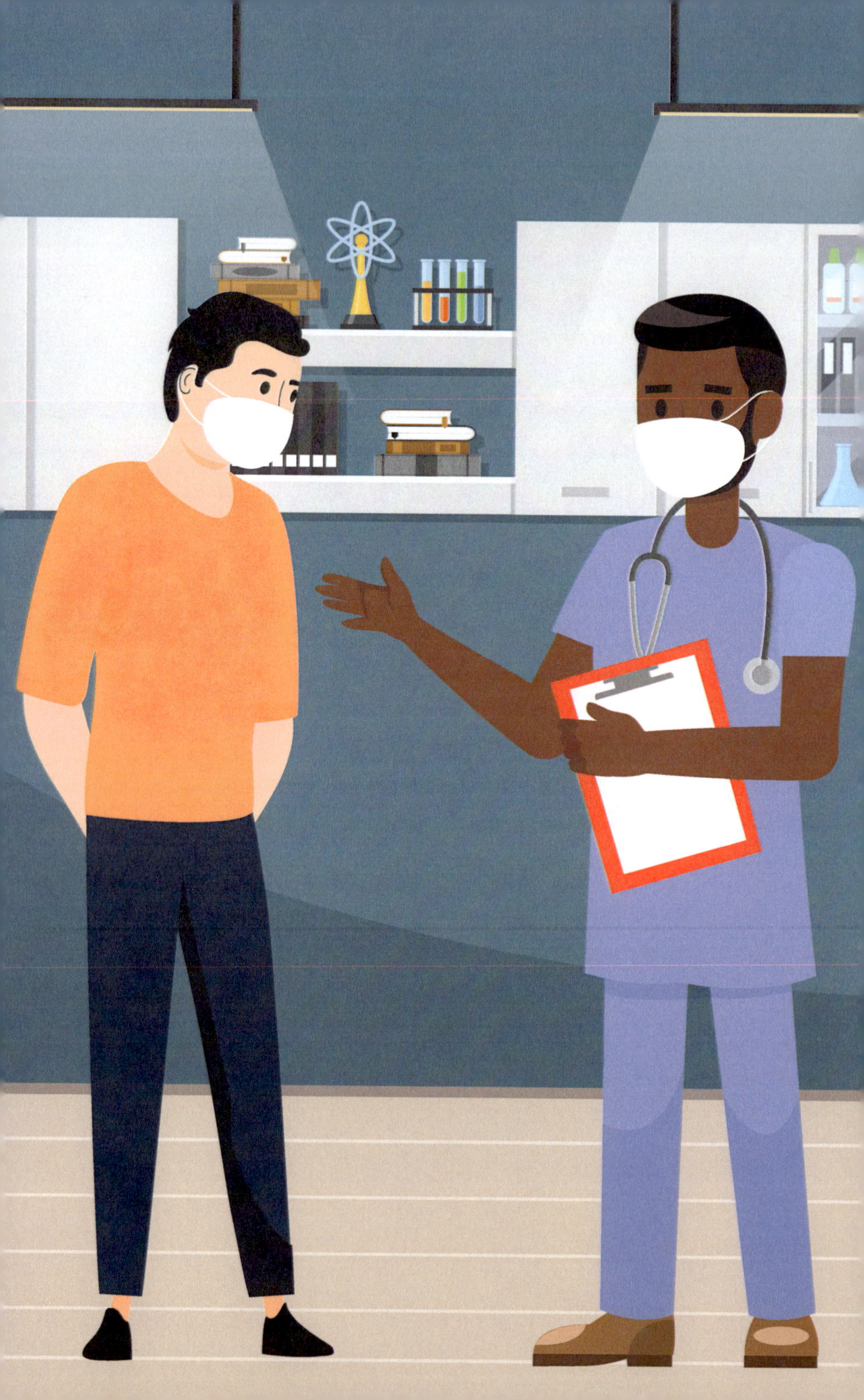

- Studying nursing theory in your free time period and understanding disease processes, pharmacology, and other theoretical concepts will help you think critically in clinical practice.

- Shadow experienced nurses on complex patient assignments. Observing how more senior nurses handle multi-disease processes and multitasking enhances your learning.

- Consider nursing externships or internship programs. These structured programs peer novice nurses with mentors and provide focused clinical experience.

- Advocate for yourself when it comes to skill practice.

- Be bold and speak up if you haven't had a chance to try a new skill and the opportunity.

- Keep an open mind and a positive attitude.

- Be receptive to constructive feedback to further your learning. Confidence will grow with experience over time.

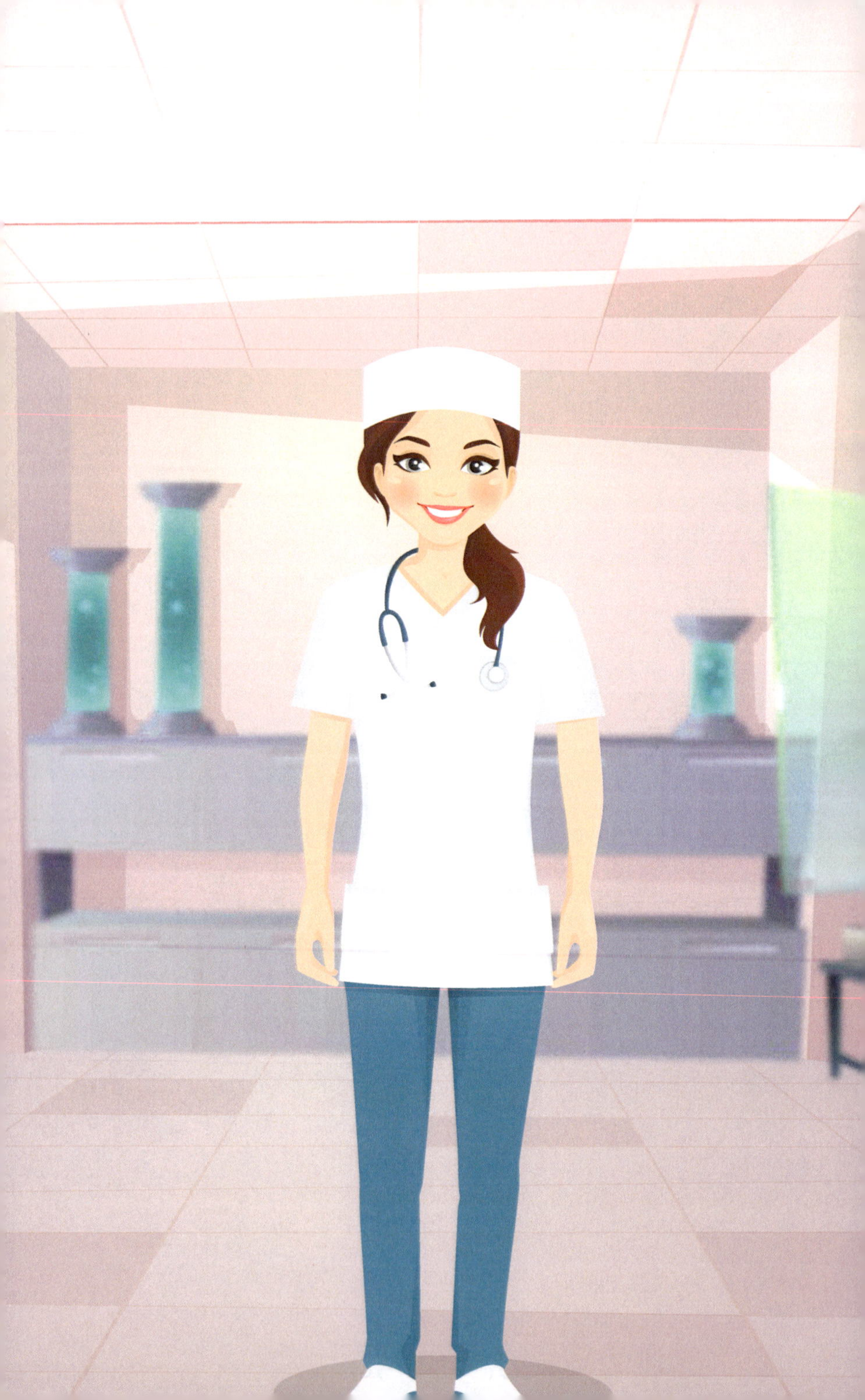

Strategies for Maintaining Composure in Emergencies

In the fast-paced world of healthcare, emergencies can strike unexpectedly, demanding swift and composed responses from nurses. Here are some comprehensive tips to help nurses understand the challenges of crisis management and decision-making:

Staying Calm Under Pressure: Strategies for Nurses

In the heat of emergencies, nurses must maintain composure.

- Mindful Breathing: Practice deep, intentional breaths to stay focused and centered.

- Prioritization Techniques: Quickly assess and prioritize tasks to address the most urgent needs first.

- Team Coordination: Collaborate efficiently with the healthcare team to distribute tasks and share responsibilities.

- Continuous Communication: Keep a clear line of communication with team members and other healthcare professionals.

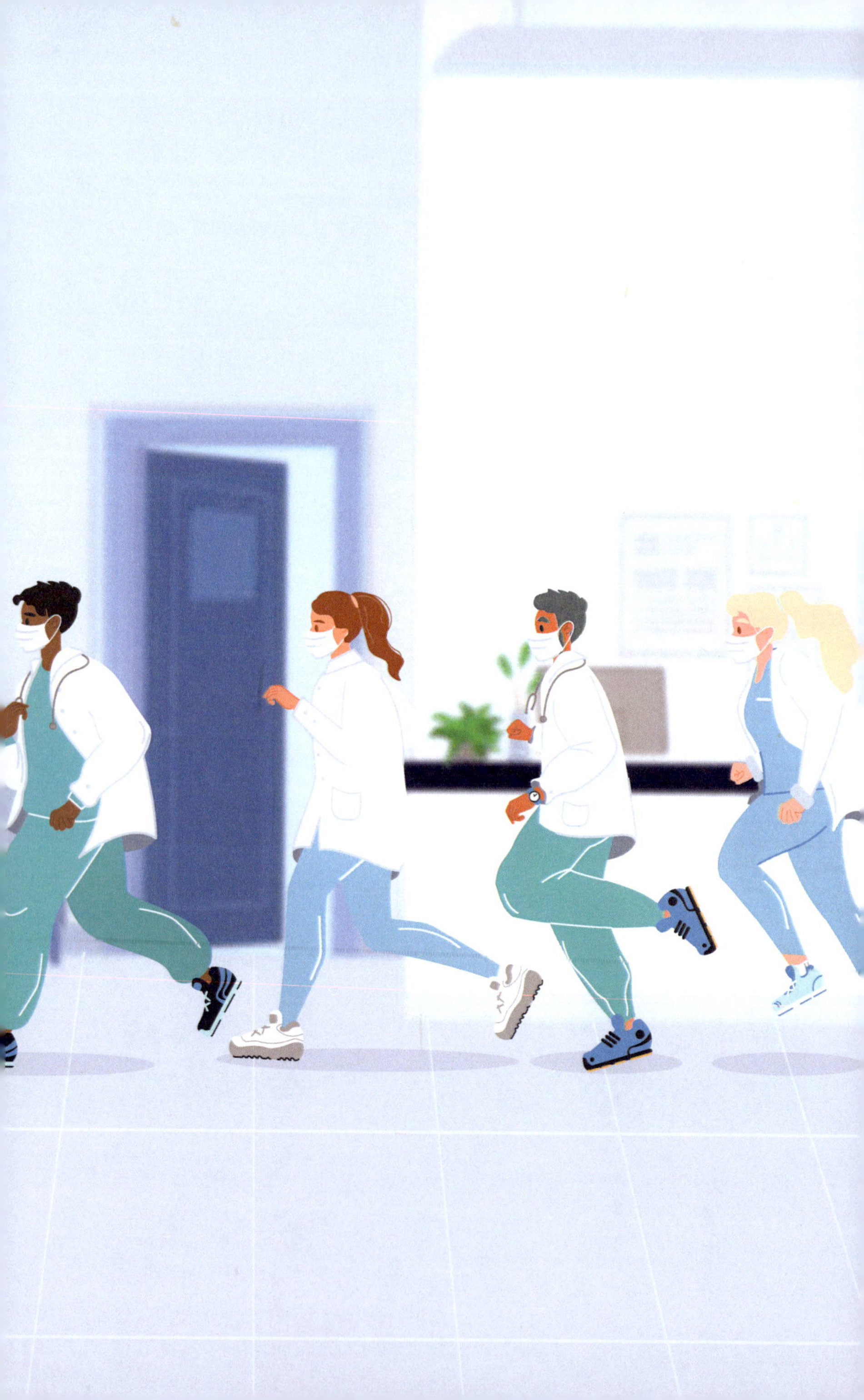

Decisive Moments: Real-Life Scenarios in Nursing

Real-life scenarios provide valuable insights into the impact of quick decision-making on patient outcomes.

- **Code Blue Response:** A nurse swiftly initiating life-saving measures during a Code Blue can be the difference between life and death.

- **Medication Errors:** Rapid identification and correction of medication errors prevent adverse reactions and enhance patient safety.

- **Timely Triage:** Effective triage decisions in a mass casualty incident can save numerous lives

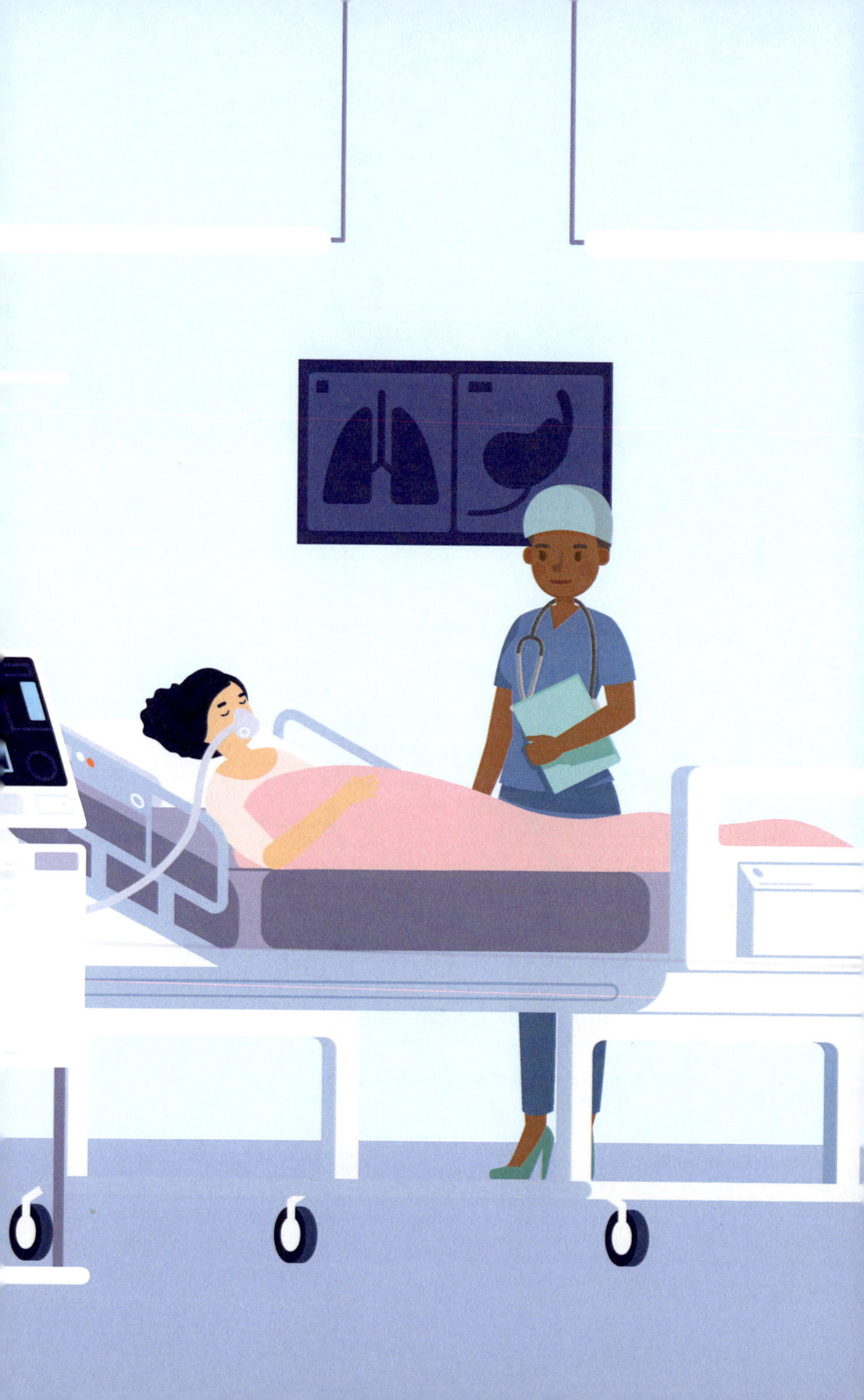

Debriefing for Growth: The Aftermath of Critical Incidents

Debriefing after critical incidents is a crucial component of personal and professional growth.

- Structured Reflection: Nurses use a structured reflection process to analyze the events and actions taken during the crisis.

- Identifying Strengths and Areas for Improvement: Debriefing helps nurses recognize their strengths and areas where further training or support may be beneficial.

- Team Learning: It fosters a culture of shared learning within the healthcare team, allowing everyone to benefit from collective experiences.

- Enhanced Resilience: Debriefing contributes to emotional resilience, helping nurses process the emotional toll of critical incidents.

With these skills in your corner, you're not just ensuring the best outcomes for your patients but creating a path for personal and professional growth. Here's to navigating the storms gracefully and embracing every opportunity for growth in your incredible nursing adventure.

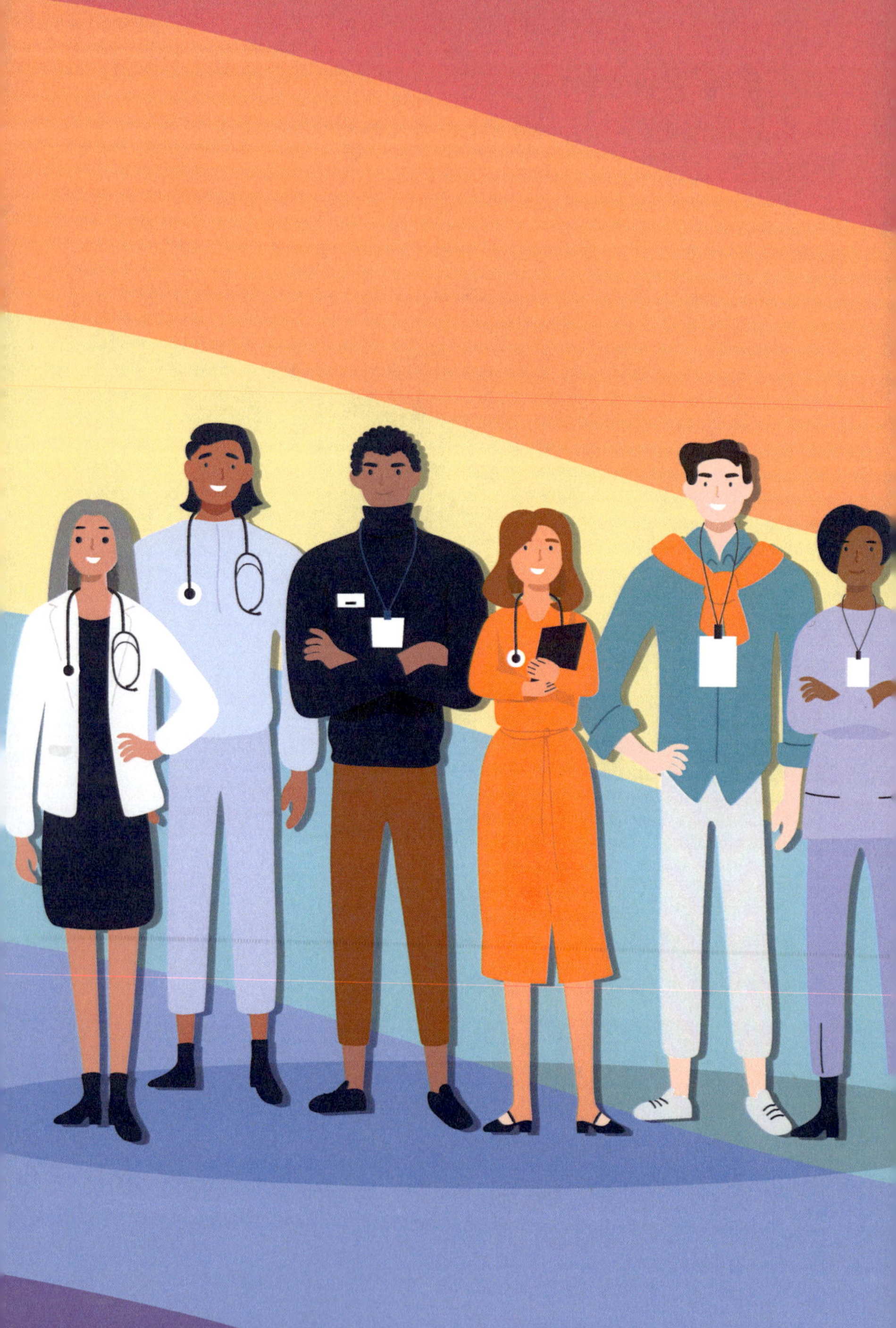

Be kind, for everyone you meet is fighting a battle." —Plato

Cultural Competence in Nursing: Embracing Diversity

Building Bridges of Understanding: Cultural Competence in Nursing

Cultural competence stands as a cornerstone for providing inclusive and effective patient care. Here's a brief tailored for nurses, illuminating the significance of cultural competence and offering practical insights:

Embracing Diversity: The Heart of Cultural Competence:

Cultural competence is not just a skill; it's an ethos that acknowledges and values the diversity of patients.

Respectful Communication: Engage with patients in a way that respects theircultural backgrounds, including language preferences andcommunication styles.

Awareness of Beliefs and Practices: Understand and appreciate the diverse beliefs, practices, and traditions that shape patients' perspectives on health and wellness.

Open-Mindedness: Cultivate an open mind, free of assumptions or stereo types, fostering an environment where patients feel understood and respected.

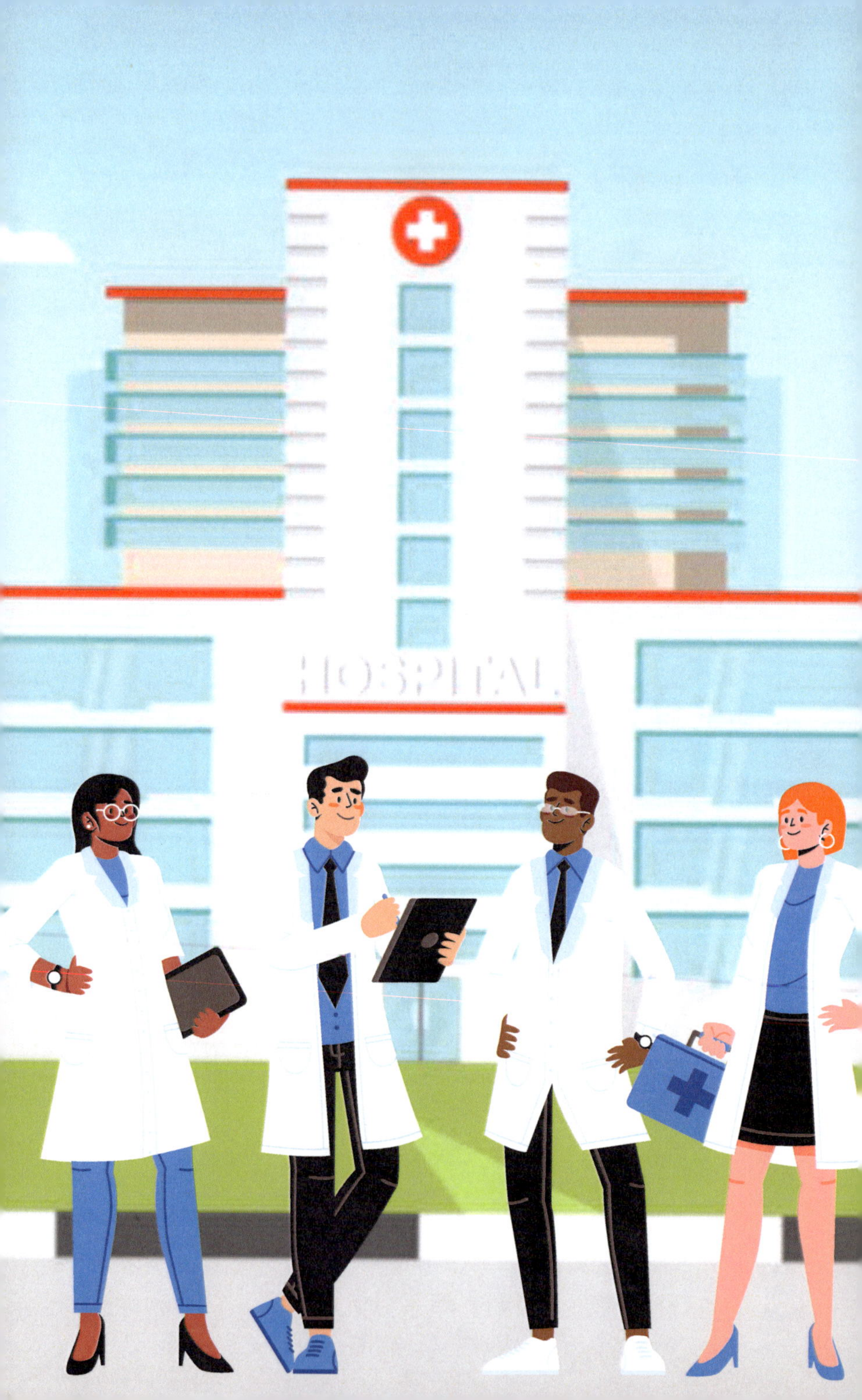
HOSPITAL

Navigating Cultural Considerations in Patient Care:

Cultural considerations can significantly impact patient care.

Treatment Preferences: Different cultures may have unique treatment modalities or intervention preferences. Family Dynamics: Cultural norms often influence family involvement in patient care decisions.

End-of-Life Practices: Understanding diverse cultural perspectives on death and end-of-life care is crucial for providing compassionate support.

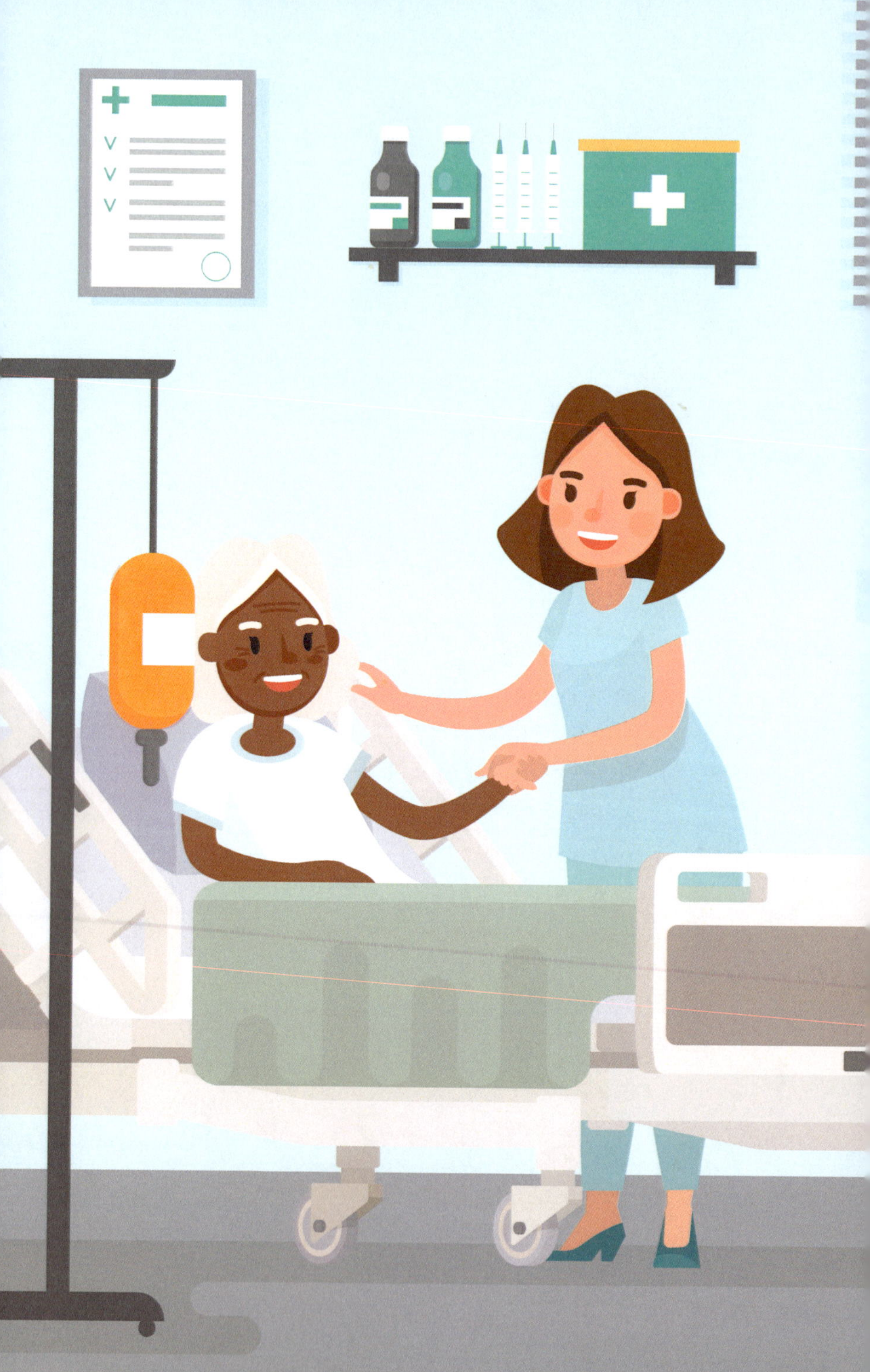

**Press forward. Do not stop or linger in your journey, but strive for the mark set before you."
-George Whitefield.**

Tips on how to Develop Effective Communication:

- Introduce yourself to patients by name and role. Say what you will be doing in a calm, reassuring manner.

- Speak clearly, make eye contact, and smile. Address patience by Mr./Mrs. or preferred name to build rapport.

- Listen actively by maintaining eye contact, nodding, and avoiding distractions. Repeat what you heard to confirm your understanding.

- Communicate in a respectful, non-judgmental manner. Be aware of tone, word choice, and potential barriers like literacy levels.

- Explain procedures and treatments in simple, easy-to-understand steps. Provide time for questions.

- Use open-ended questions to elicit full details from patients about concerns, pain level, etcetera.

- When reporting to other staff, include relevant assessment findings, changes in condition, and actions taken succinctly and organized.

- Document in an objective, factual way without abbreviations.

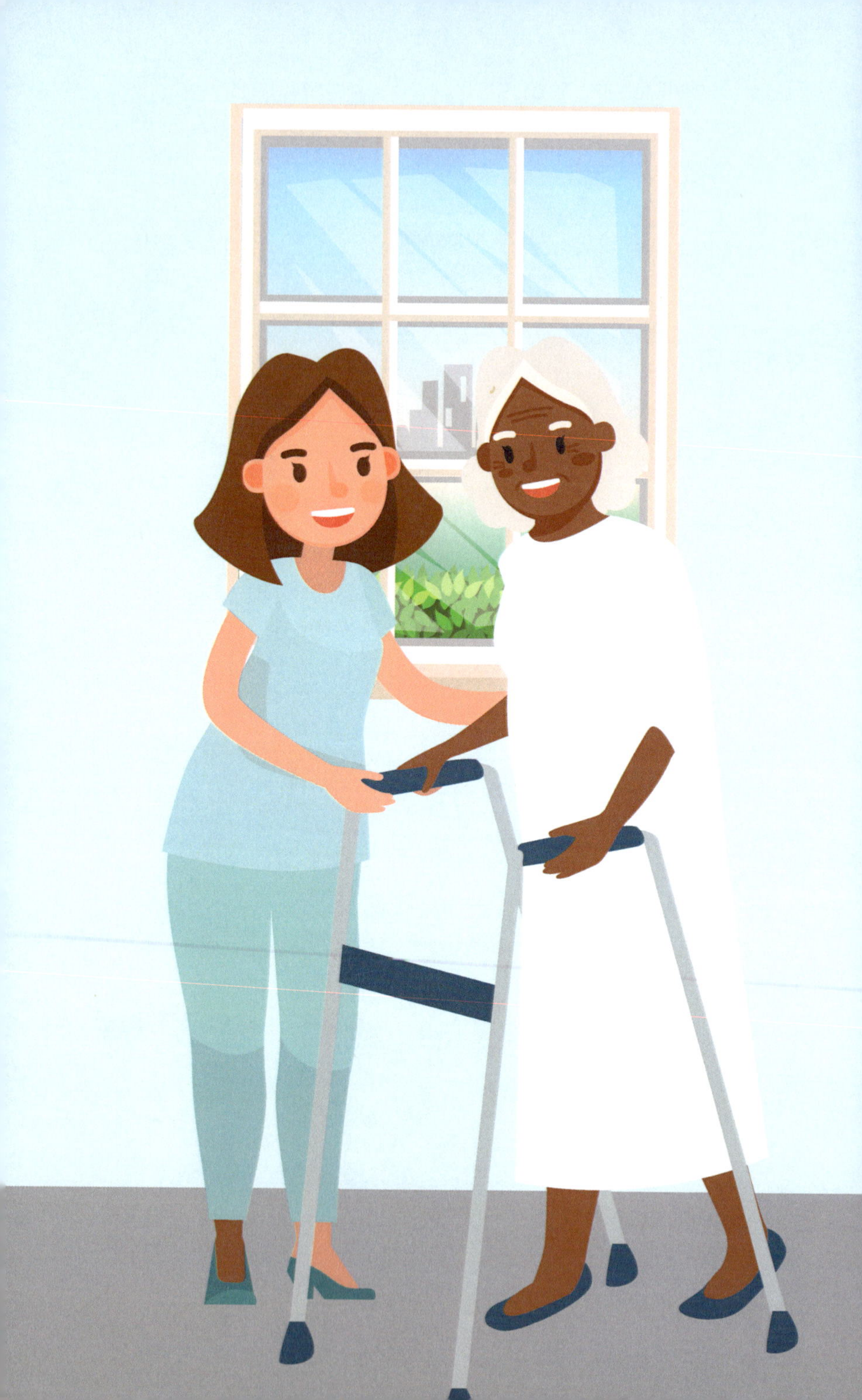

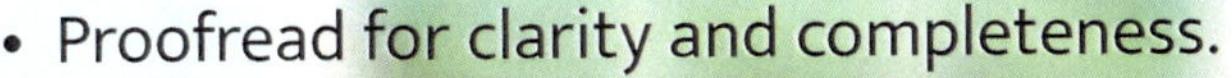

- Proofread for clarity and completeness.

- Communicate assertively by making eye contact, speaking firmly, and providing context for requests.

- Participate in handoff huddles and be proactive in communicating patient concerns across shifts.

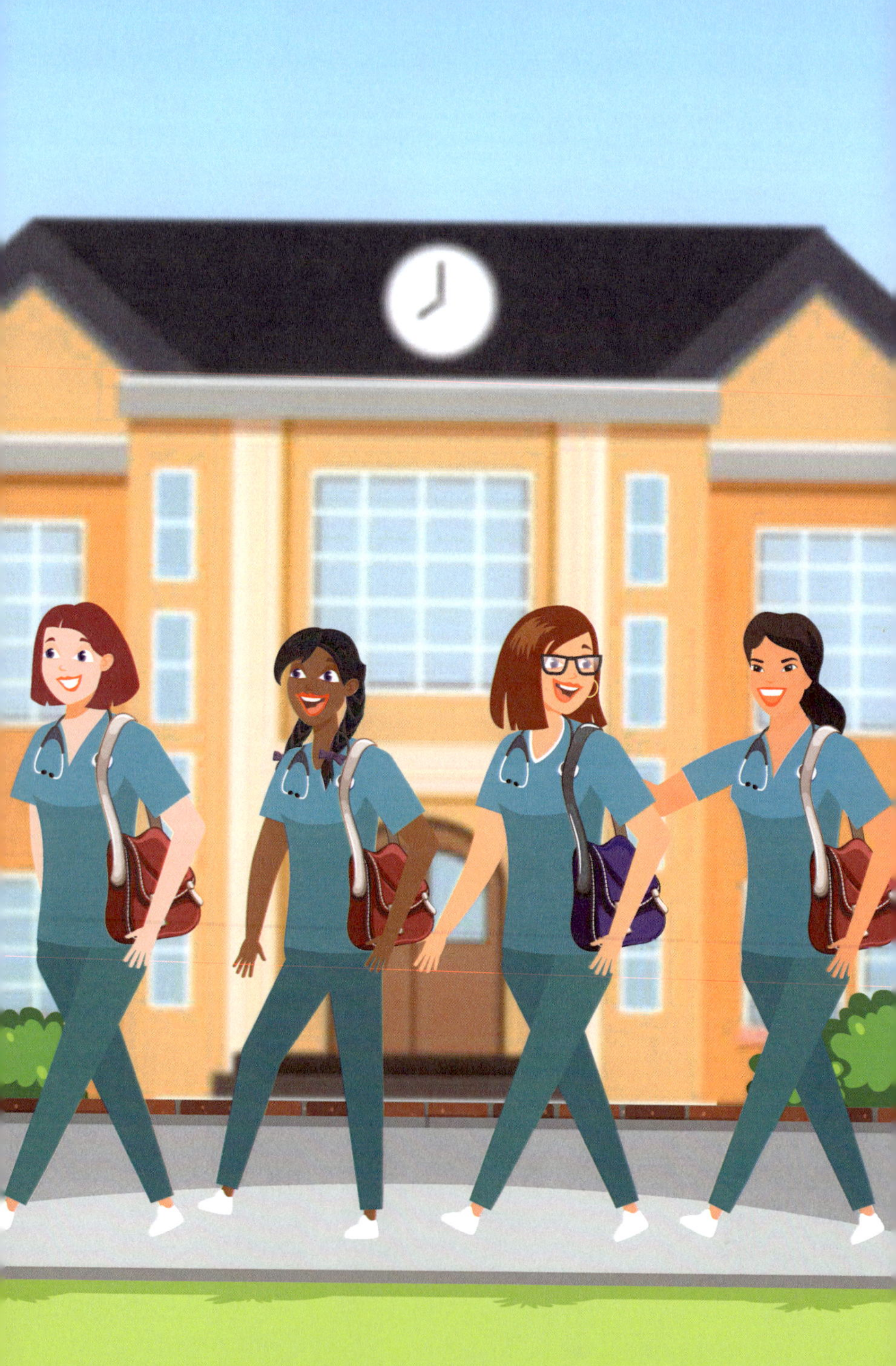

Resources and Training Opportunities for Enhanced Competence:

Empower nurses with resources and training opportunities to fortify their cultural competence.

Cultural Competence Workshops: Encourage participation in workshops that delve into cultural awareness, humility, and effective cross- cultural communication.

Online Modules and Courses: Provide access to online resources that offer in-depth cultural competency training.

Diverse Reading Materials: Recommend literature that explores various cultural perspectives, fostering a deeperunderstanding of diverse traditions and values.

By embracing cultural competence, nurses enrich their practice and contribute to a healthcare environment where every patient feels heard, valued, and understood. It's not just about treating illnesses; it's about honoring the unique tapestry of every individual under your care.

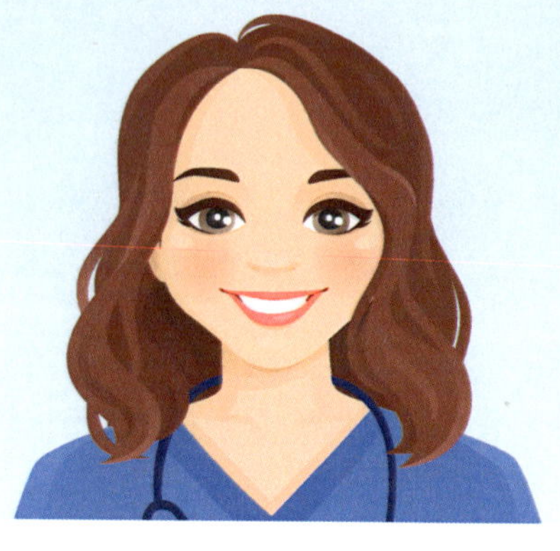
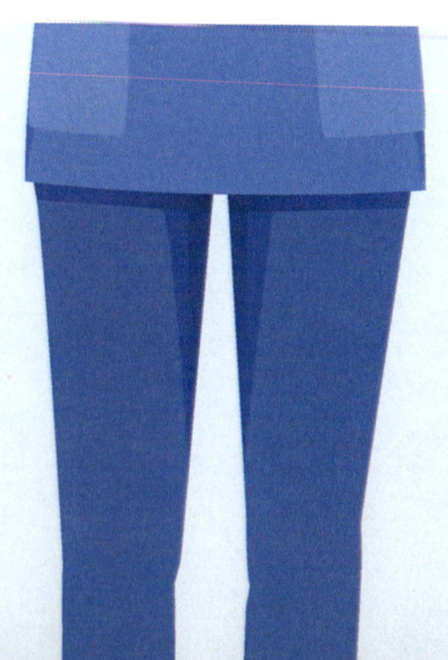

ETHIC

Nurse: just another word to describe a person strong enough to tolerate anything and soft enough to understand anyone." — Unknown

Ethical Dilemmas and Nursing Ethics

Charting the Course Through Ethical Waters: A Nurse's Compass

Ethical dilemmas are inevitable; nurses often find themselves at the crossroads of tough decisions. Let's dive deeper into how you can get through these hurdles.

Common Ethical Dilemmas: Navigating the Gray Areas

Ethical dilemmas come in various forms, and nurses must adeptly navigate them.

Patient Autonomy vs. Beneficence: Balancing a patient's right to autonomy with the imperative to do good.

Resource Allocation: Deciding how to distribute limited resources ethically.

Truthfulness and Informed Consent: Striking a balance between truthfulness and respecting a patient's autonomy in decision-making.

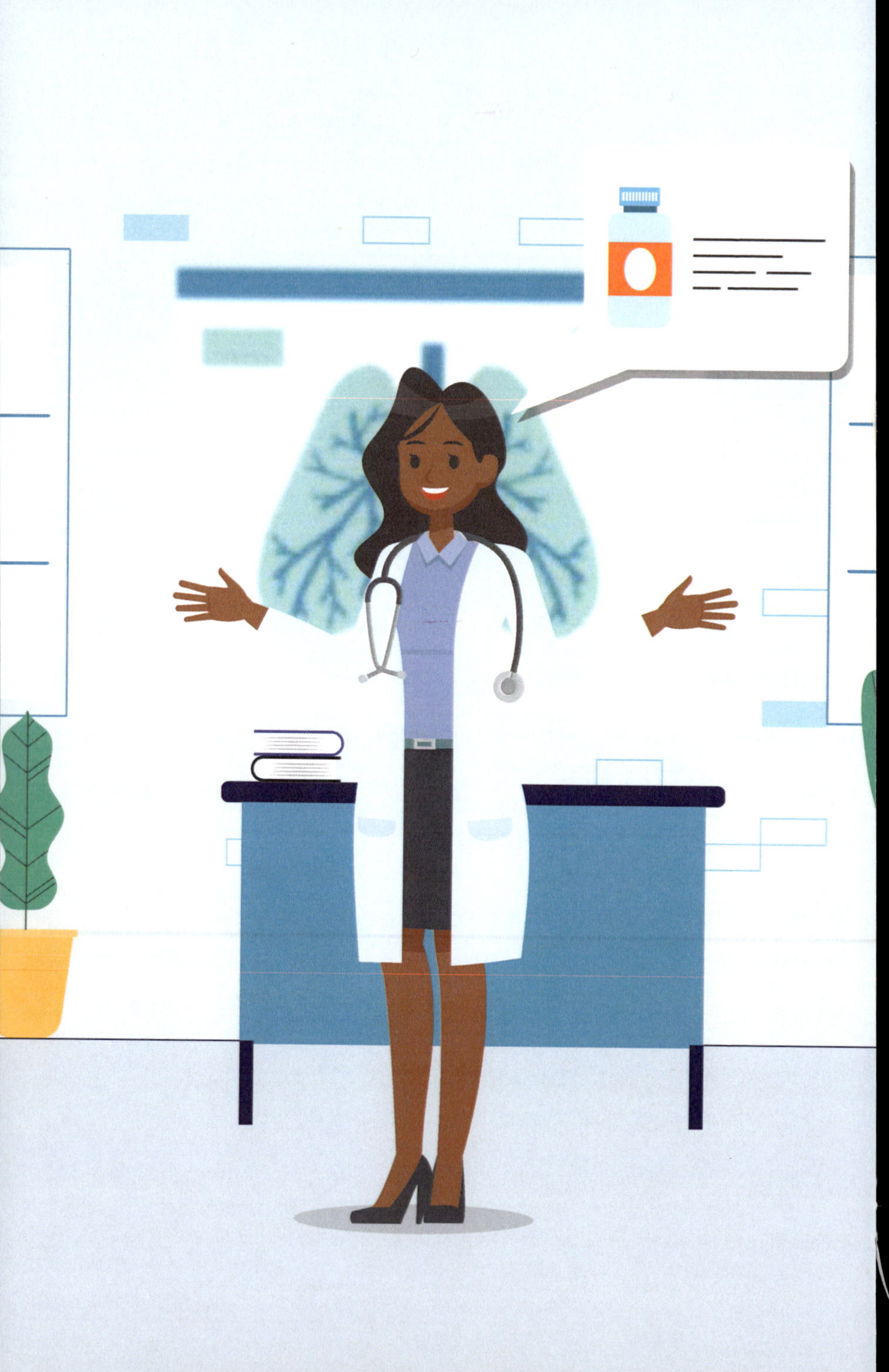

The Nursing Code of Ethics: A Moral Compass in Daily Practice

Delve into the nursing code of ethics as the moral compass guiding nurses through daily practice.

Advocacy: Emphasize the nurse's role as a patient advocate, ensuring their rights and wishes are upheld.

Accountability: Discuss the importance of accountability in ethical decision-making, focusing on taking responsibility for one's actions.

Professional Boundaries: Explore the nuances of maintaining professional boundaries to ensure ethical practice.

Ethical Decision-Making Frameworks: Tools for Clarity

Equipping nurses with practical frameworks and tools to aid in ethical decision-making.

The Four Principles Approach: Applying the principles of autonomy, beneficence, non-maleficence, and justice to ethical dilemmas.

The Ethical Decision-Making Model: A systematic process involving identifying the problem, considering alternatives, and making an informed decision.

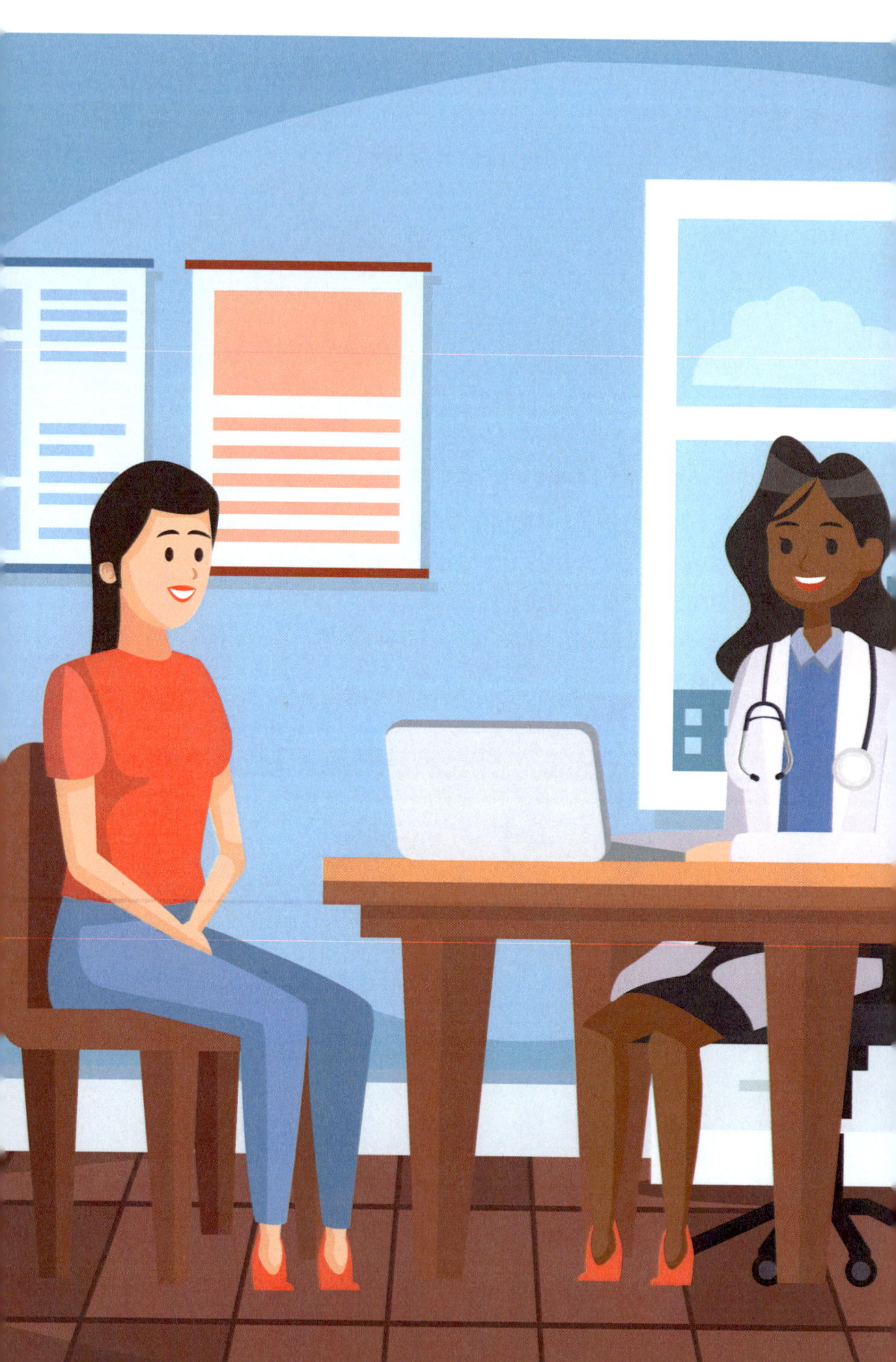

Consultation and Collaboration: Encouraging nurses to seek input from colleagues, ethics committees, and other professionals to ensure a comprehensive perspective. It's not just about your decisions; it's about building trust and ensuring that every bit of care you provide meets the gold standard of ethical excellence.

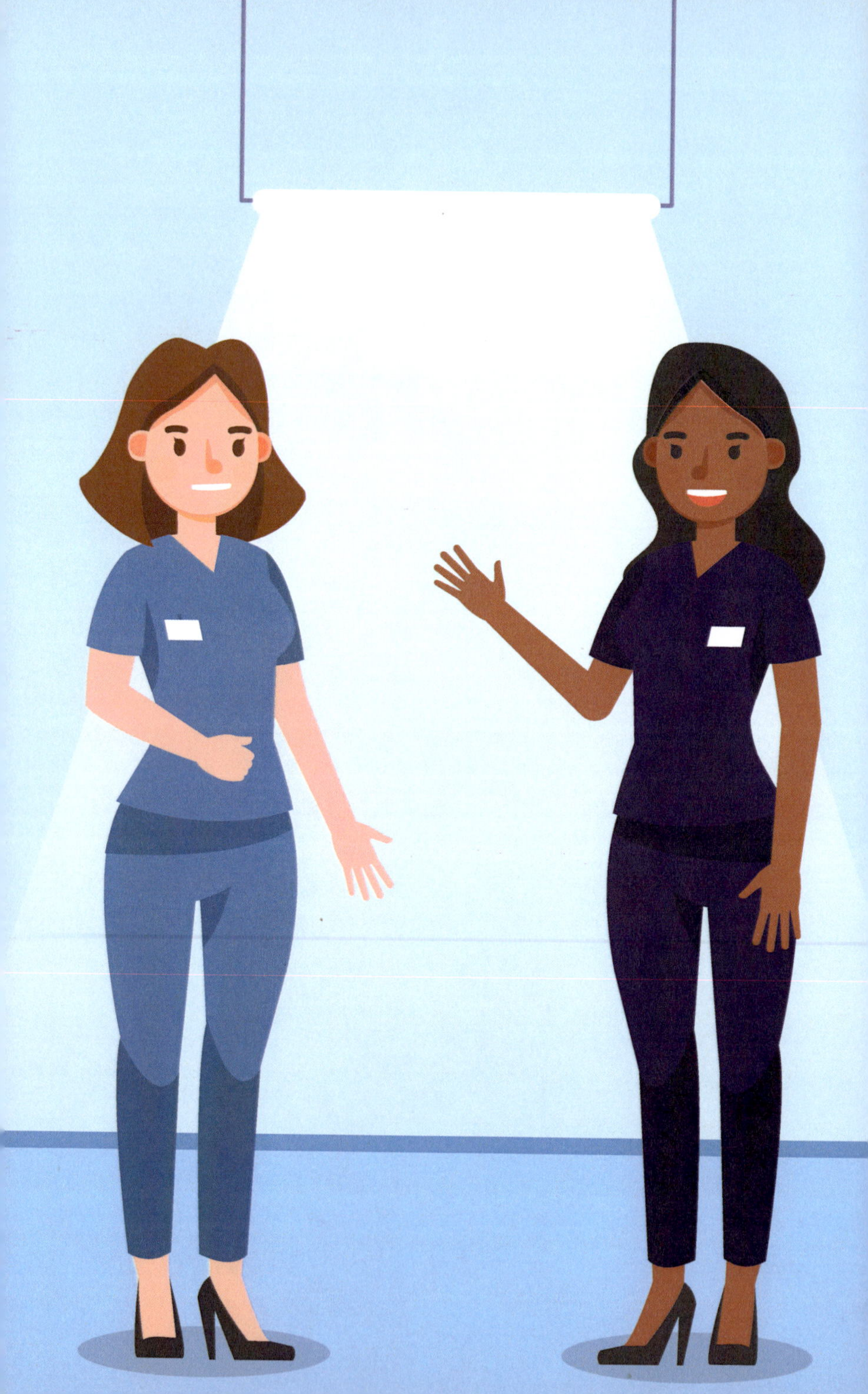

Mentoring is a brain to pick, an ear to listen, and a push in the right direction."- John C. Crosby.

A Pathway to Discovering a Mentor

In the expansive and dynamic nursing field, the progression from novice to seasoned professional is enhanced through the insights and direction experienced mentors provide. Here is a list of factors that you need to take into consideration:

Observation in the Workplace
Initiate your exploration by keenly observing the experienced nurses in your immediate work environment or clinical setting.

Identify Role Models
Pinpoint individuals whose wealth of expertise aligns harmoniously with your envisioned career trajectory.

Evaluate Patient Care Approaches
Scrutinize and discern the approaches seasoned nurses employ in their patient care methodologies.

Align Career Aspirations
Look for professionals whose career journeys and accomplishments mirror your aspirations in nursing.

Seek Resonance
Identify those whose patient care approach resonates with your values, creating a meaningful connection.

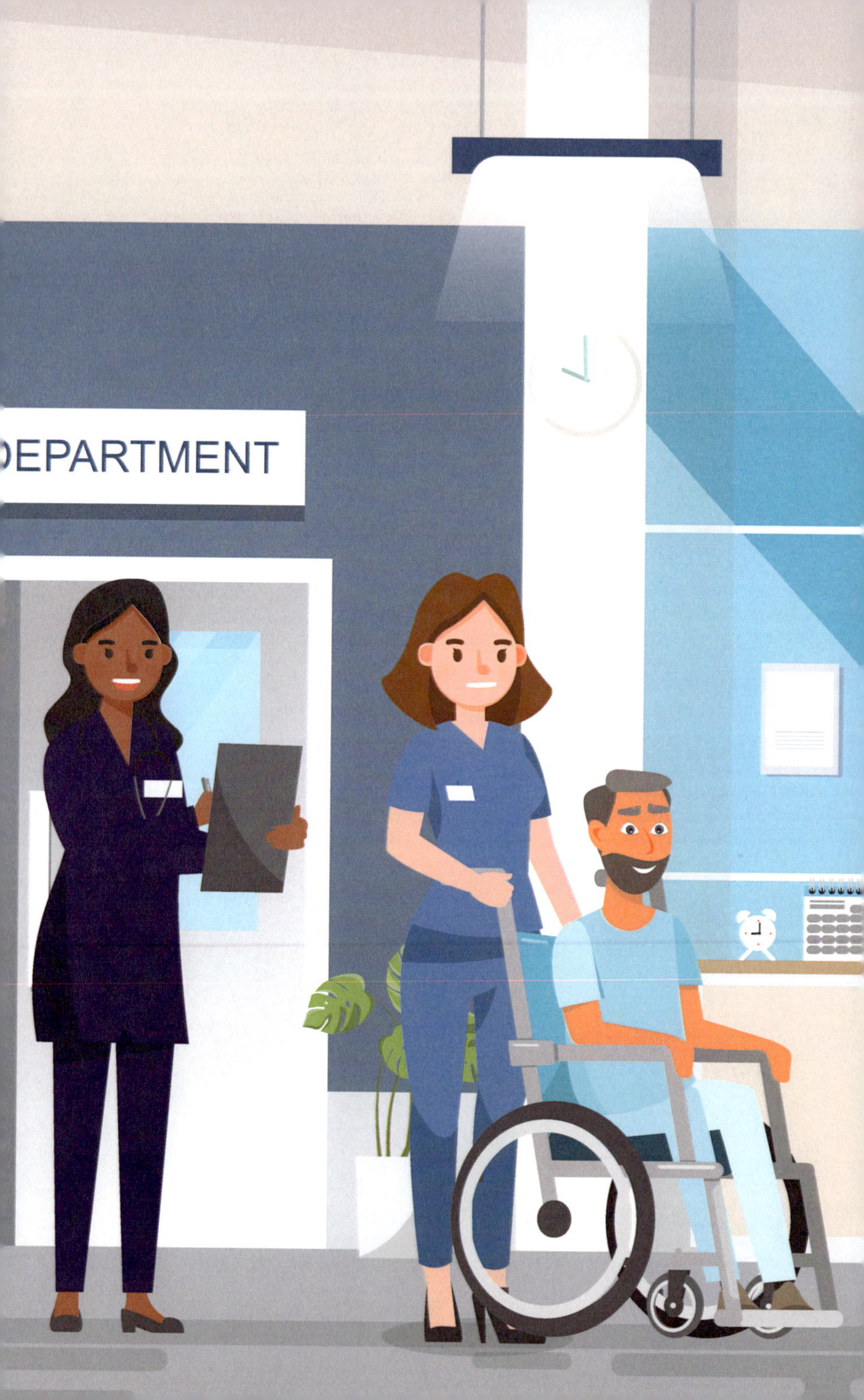
DEPARTMENT

Consider Diverse Roles
Broaden your scope by considering nurses in various roles, such as charge nurses, nursing educators, or specialized practitioners.

Look Beyond Job Titles
Explore beyond formal titles; seek out individuals whose practical insights and daily contributions embody the essence of nursing excellence.

Consider Institutional Leaders
Extend your observations to include nurse leaders or administrators who may provide a broader perspective on the nursing profession.

Extend Observation to Clinical Rotations
Expand your watchful eye during clinical rotations to identify mentors among healthcare professionals who demonstrate exemplary nursing practices.

Build a Diverse Network
Establish connections with a diverse array of seasoned professionals, ensuring a comprehensive understanding of various facets of the nursing landscape.

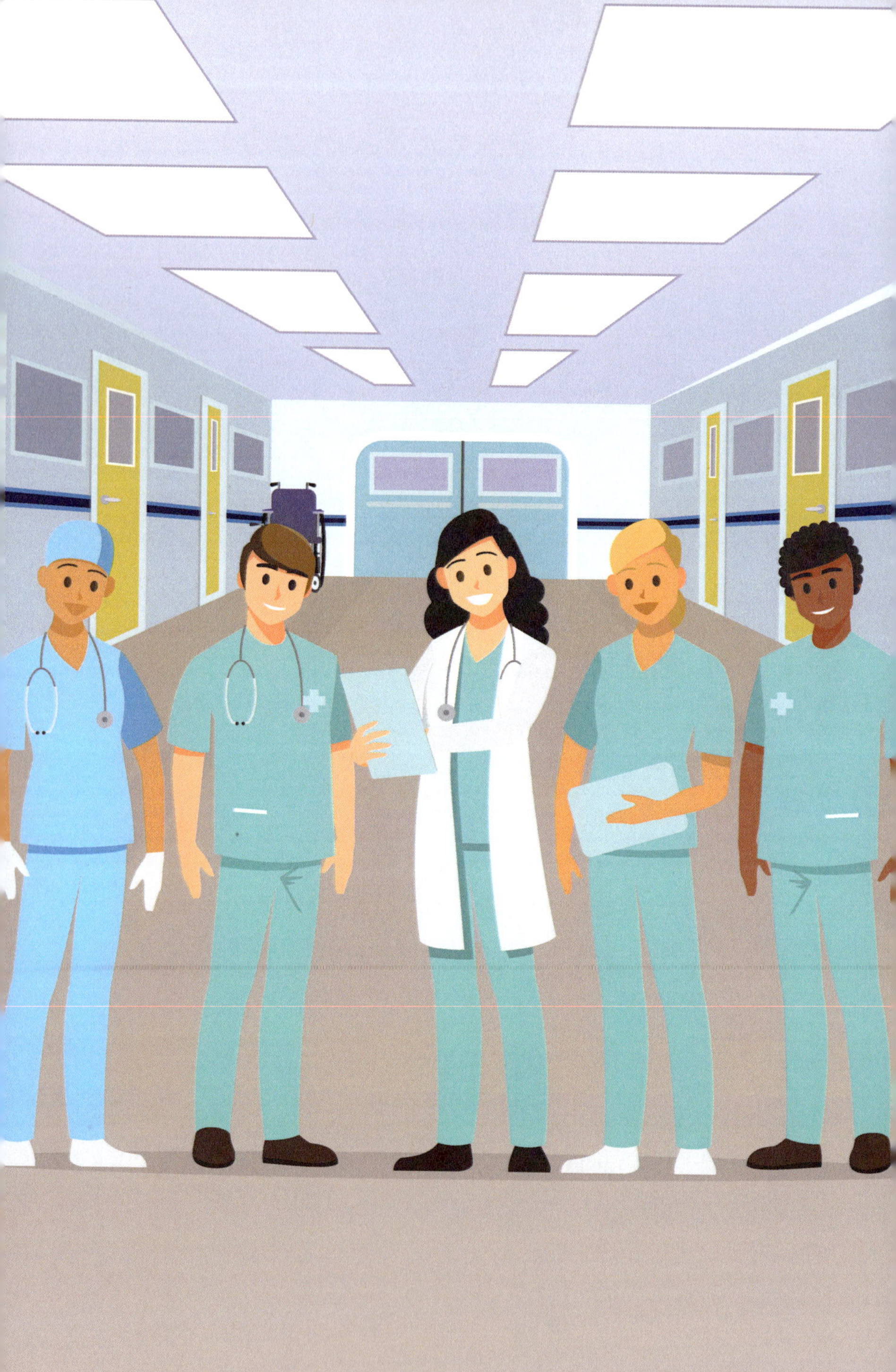

Seek opportunities to interact with nurse leaders and administrators. These individuals often carry a wealth of experience and can provide insights into clinical practice, l eadership, and career advancement.

Identify Networking Opportunities
Actively seek events, conferences, or professional gatherings where nurse leaders and administrators may be present.

Attend Leadership Forums
Participate in leadership-focused forums, workshops, or seminars to connect with nurse leaders who share their insights and experiences.

Utilize Professional Organizations
Engage with nursing associations or organizations that attract nurse leaders. Attend meetings and events to facilitate meaningful connections.

Explore Internal Workshops
Inquire about internal workshops or training sessions where nurse leaders may participate in your healthcare institution.

Leverage Online Platforms
Utilize online platforms, forums, or social media groups dedicated to nursing leadership. Engage in discussions and seek guidance from experienced nurse leaders.

Request Informational Interviews
Approach nurse leaders for informational interviews, expressing your interest in learning from their experiences in both clinical practice and leadership roles.

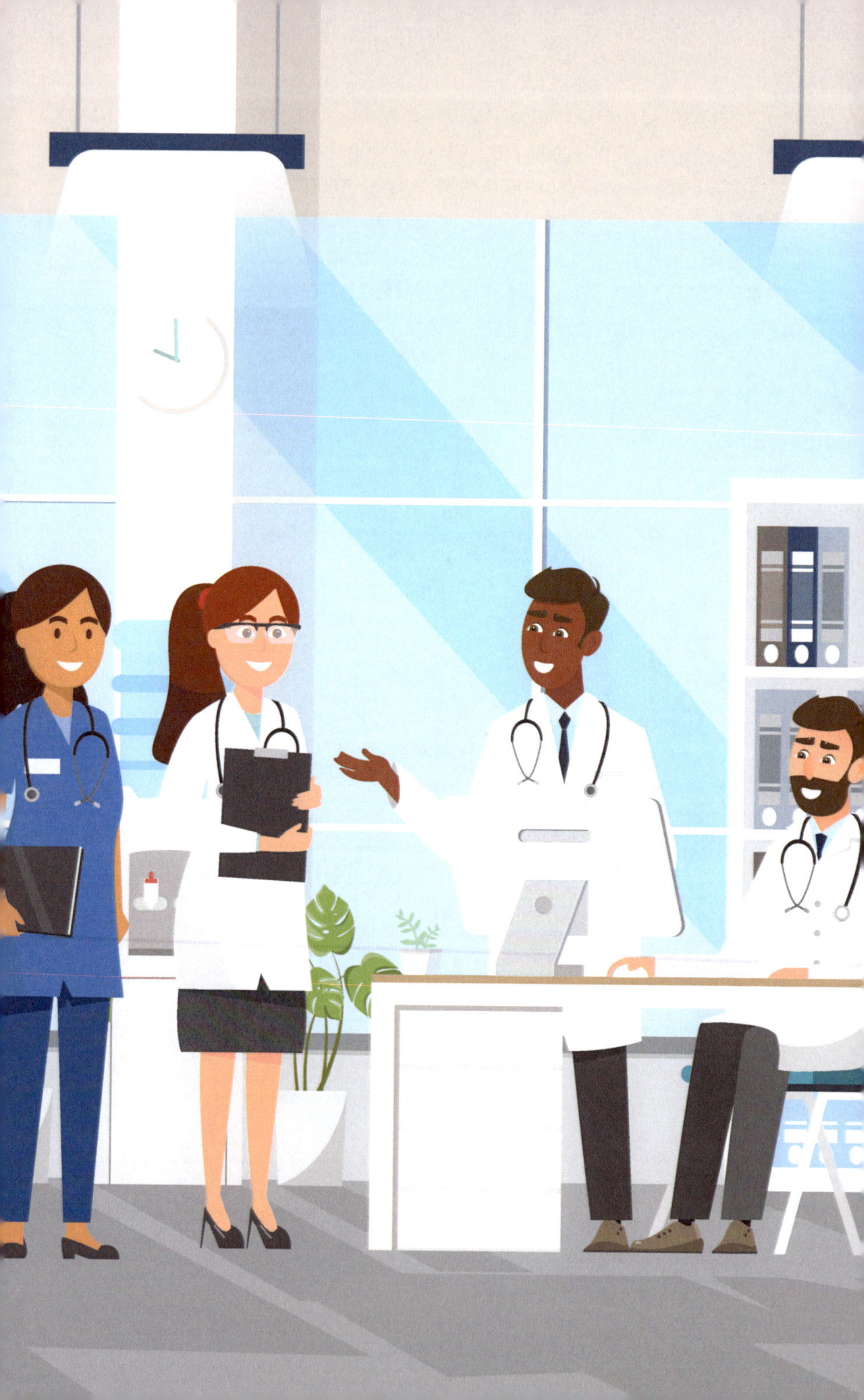

Participate in Mentorship Programs
Enroll in mentorship programs that specifically pair nurses with experienced leaders. These programs often provide structured opportunities for interaction.

Seek Guidance on Career Advancement
Pose thoughtful questions to nurse leaders regarding their career progression and insights on navigating the path to leadership roles.

Attend Administrative Meetings
Attend administrative meetings within your healthcare institution to observe and connect with nurse leaders whenever feasible.

Express Interest in Mentorship
Communicate your interest in mentorship to nurse leaders, showcasing your eagerness to learn and grow under their guidance.

Remember, this guide is a compass, not a map. Just like our fingerprints, our journeys, paths, challenges, and victories are different. You may encounter different things, but your compassion, resilience, and thirst for knowledge will pave the road. Wishing you fair winds and following seas, dear nurse, on your journey towards growth and wisdom.

NOTES

NOTES

NOTES

NOTES

NOTES